INTERPERSONAL
PSYCHOTHERAPY FOR GROUP

INTERPERSONAL PSYCHOTHERAPY FOR GROUP

Denise E. Wilfley, Ph.D.
K. Roy MacKenzie, M.D.
R. Robinson Welch, Ph.D.
Virginia E. Ayres, Ph.D.
Myrna M. Weissman, Ph.D.

BASIC
BOOKS

A Member of the Perseus Books Group

Published by Basic Books,
A Member of the Perseus Books Group

Library of Congress Cataloging-in-Publication Data

Interpersonal psychology for group / Denise E. Wilfley ... [et.al]
    p. cm. -- (Basic behavioral science)
  Includes bibliographical references and index.
  ISBN 0-465-09569-0
    1. Interpersonal psychotherapy.   I. Wilfley, Denise., 1960- II. Series.

RC489.I55 I584 2000
616.89'14--dc21   99-086316

FIRST EDITION

00 01 02 03 / 10 9 8 7 6 5 4 3 2 1

To my parents, Arlene and Donald Wilfley,
my brother and sisters, nephews and nieces, who have
given the gifts of connection and a sense of belonging to me
—DEW

To my parents, Reuben and Mary Jo Welch,
my sister, Susan, and to my late uncle,
Charles Welch, whose life was a testament to
the sustaining power of interpersonal relationships.
—RRW

To my mother, Beverly J. Morcheid,
my family and friends.
—VA

To my husband, the late Gerald L. Klerman,
who originated IPT.
—MMW

Contents

Acknowledgments

We would like to express our gratitude to the many individuals who have made this project possible:

We are indebted to the hundreds of patients who have been willing to share their lives with us and have given us the opportunity to experience with them, in the context of IPT-G, the remarkable changes in their interpersonal lives. We would also like to thank those colleagues and mentors who have skillfully taught us and pushed our thinking forward about IPT—Cleon Cornes, M.D., Ellen Frank, Ph.D., Gay Herrington, Ph.D., the late Gerald L. Klerman, M.D., Mary Beth Rauktis, Ph.D., and Bruce J. Rounsaville, M.D. The authors are thankful to the universities that have supported the work on IPT and IPT-G—Stanford University, Yale University, San Diego State University, Columbia College of Physicians and Surgeons, and Cornell Medical School. We also thank the National Institutes of Health, specifically the National Institute of Mental Health for providing funding for the efficacy studies of IPT-G with binge eating disorder. We are also grateful to those therapists and research colleagues who, by never-ending dedication and hard work, have helped refine and breathe life into the treatment and into this manual—Susan Beren, Ph. D., Lisa M. Cohen, Ph.D., Mary Ann Frank, Ph.D., and Emily Borman Spurrell, Ph.D. Finally, there are a number of individuals who have worked diligently behind the scenes to ensure the accuracy and quality of this manuscript—Paul Cavazos, Kelli Glass, and Danielle Kukene. Special thanks to Sarah Aronson, M.D., for her endless support and her insightful comments on earlier revisions of this manuscript, and to Elizabeth Barber and Denise Abraham for their rigorous proofreading and editing of this manuscript.

Preface

This book originated in 1989 while Denise Wilfley was beginning a postdoctoral fellowship in behavioral medicine within the Department of Psychiatry at Stanford University. During that year, Wilfley and her colleagues began developing a research protocol designed to compare cognitive-behavior therapy (CBT) and interpersonal psychotherapy (IPT) for the treatment of nonpurging bulimia nervosa (now known as binge eating disorder, or BED), using group as the intervention modality. Although CBT had been used widely in groups, to date there had never been a group adaptation of IPT. As luck would have it, Wilfley's office at Stanford was across from that of Irvin D. Yalom, M.D., who consulted with Wilfley about adapting IPT to a group. Wilfley's work at Stanford resulted in the first IPT-G manual as well as completion of the first empirical study of IPT-G, which was published in 1993 while Wilfley was at Yale. During her years at Yale, Wilfley worked closely with Bruce Rounsaville, M.D., one of the originators of IPT, to refine the adaptation of IPT to group. Roy MacKenzie's involvement in this project began in June 1995 at the annual meeting of the Society for Psychotherapy Research in Vancouver, B.C. MacKenzie posted a notice asking if anyone knew of others who were developing the use of IPT in a group format. An anonymous responder identified Denise Wilfley. This fortuitous contact grew into regular correspondence, culminating in an initial brainstorming session between MacKenzie, Wilfley, and Robinson Welch in 1996 at Yale. Later that year, during the American Psychiatric Association meeting in New York City, Wilfley and MacKenzie met with Myrna Weissman. Then, in 1997, during the American Psychiatric Association meeting in San Diego, a final organizational meeting was attended by the present authors. The planning of the current manual for IPT-G began at this time.

To this manual Denise Wilfley brings an extensive research background and a series of major published studies concerning the treatment of eating disorders, particularly binge eating disorder. Much of this research has involved comparative studies of IPT and CBT. Roy MacKenzie has published widely concerning the theory and practice of group psychotherapy, particularly the use of time-limited models. MacKenzie was trained in the delivery of IPT by Cleon Cornes, M.D., who was the lead IPT trainer for the NIMH collaborative depression project. MacKenzie's clinical work centers on the group treatment of patients with major depression. He is currently conducting a clinical effectiveness study using IPT-G for treatment-resistant depression. These two clinical areas—eating disorders and major depression—represent a significant component of mental health service delivery systems; they also involve syndromes for which group approaches have historically been used in treatment. Wilfley's studies have established the efficacy of IPT-G for binge eating disorder, and MacKenzie's clinical effectiveness study of seven IPT-G groups for treatment-resistant depression is promising but requires further corroboration.

Rob Welch began working with Wilfley on the initial IPT-G manual in the late 1980s. In 1991, he became the lead IPT-G therapist on Wilfley's recently completed NIMH comparative trial of group CBT and IPT-G for BED. Over the last ten years, Welch has worked closely with Wilfley on the continued refinement and delivery of IPT-G. To the present book he brings his extensive clinical and research experience in the delivery of IPT-G.

Virginia Ayres has broad experience in the application of IPT in both clinical and research settings. Trained by Dr. Cornes, Ayres initially garnered experience in the practice of individual IPT for patients with recurrent major depression in research settings where she worked with Ellen Frank, Ph.D. Ayres's involvement in the current project began after she attended an IPT-G workshop given by Denise

Wilfley and Rob Welch in 1995. Ayres trained with Wilfley and Welch in the delivery of IPT-G and subsequently conducted open research studies in the community using IPT-G for women with binge eating disorder. Her experience with group and individual IPT in the treatment of eating disorders and major depression has provided depth and clarity to the development of this manual.

Myrna Weissman provides a crucial connection: the origins of interpersonal therapy. Along with her late husband, Gerald L. Klerman, M.D., Weissman was intimately involved in IPT's development and refinement. Her involvement and extensive dedication to IPT in research projects and in numerous controlled clinical trials continue to this day. Indeed, her vast experience with IPT has been of great value to the preparation of this manual. Thanks in large part to Weissman, IPT has steadily gained in status over the last decade as an effective treatment for major depression and an increasing array of other syndromes.

The clinical examples used in this book are drawn from clinical populations exhibiting both eating disorders and mood disorders. As such, these examples address not only the impulsivity and affect management that characterize the eating disorders but also the inhibition/social withdrawal and cognitive deficits associated with major depression. All case material has been substantially altered so as to prevent any discernible connection between clinical vignettes and the actual patients treated.

IPT is based on a rich tradition of interpersonal theory and meticulous clinical research, and group psychotherapy shares much of this tradition. Moreover, a substantial empirical database indicates that the effectiveness of group psychotherapy is equal to that of individual psychotherapy across a wide range of models and disorders. The exciting challenge of this book, then, has been to seize the opportunity to systematically bring together these various clinical sources. Groups, by their very nature, are interpersonal and form a natural delivery platform on which to apply the strategies of IPT. In the hope of encouraging further studies in this area, the authors make passing references throughout to other emerging uses of IPT-G that have not yet been subject to empirical evaluation.

Another incentive for this book is related to the increasing importance placed on the use of the group modality in service systems. The authors share the concern that pressure for the use of this modality has been driven in large part by the cost-effectiveness of time-limited groups. Indeed, as the number of sessions is often very limited in such groups and their membership is continuously changing, even if IPT concepts are used the restricted format precludes the intensive psychotherapy goal of IPT. We have tried to address this concern by being very clear about the structure of the frame of therapy. We have also placed considerable emphasis on the assessment and preparation of patients for IPT-G. This approach goes somewhat beyond that described in the individual-IPT manual, although we believe it is quite congruent with the spirit of that publication. As a pregroup procedure, it is designed to create a clear set of target goals that are subsumed beneath the IPT "problem areas." And as our clinical experience has indicated, it is a helpful method of maintaining a focus within the complexity of group interaction.

The empirical support for IPT-G is strongest within the eating disorder population, as the careful comparative studies conducted by Denise Wilfley and her colleagues make abundantly clear. It is our hope that the publication of this manual will serve as an incentive for clinical researchers to begin broadening the scope of empirically supported applications of IPT-G, as has already occurred in the case of IPT. To our knowledge, four studies utilizing our group adaptation of IPT are now under way: Josh Lipzit and his colleagues at Columbia University have adapted IPT-G for social phobia, Janice Krupnick at Georgetown University has further adapted IPT-G for abused women with acute posttraumatic stress disorder (PTSD), Laura Mufson is currently adapting IPT-G in the treatment of adolescent depression, and Geraldine Dowse in New Zealand has adapted IPT-G for use with patients recently diagnosed with cancer.

Above all, this book is directed to the practicing clinician. IPT is a safe, focused model that serves as an ideal vehicle for implementing the common factors underlying all of the psychotherapies. At the same time, the intensive interactional group format provides a powerful mix of interpersonal support and interpersonal challenge that encourages participants to become involved and motivated. The treatment approach we propose, which combines the IPT model and the group modality, provides a cost-effective time-limited protocol within which the clinician has flexibility to apply a range of effective techniques. It also offers an intensive psychotherapeutic experience that fits the needs of patients with such difficult and persistent syndromes as major depression and eating disorders.

PART ONE
INTRODUCTION, BACKGROUND, AND THEORY

CHAPTER 1

Interpersonal Psychotherapy: Background, Concepts, and Adaptation to Group

EMPIRICAL AND THEORETICAL FRAMEWORKS OF IPT

EMPIRICAL BASIS FOR IPT

Interpersonal psychotherapy (IPT) is a brief, time-limited psychotherapy that was initially developed for the treatment of nonbipolar, nonpsychotic depressed outpatients. The full details of the method and the theoretical, strategic, and empirical issues involved were first published in Klerman, Weissman, Rounsaville, and Chevron (1984). A comprehensive update can now be found in Weissman, et al. (2000). Clinicians interested in applying the group model (IPT-G) outlined in this book are encouraged to obtain training in IPT, as outlined in the new comprehensive guide.

IPT has demonstrated efficacy for the treatment of several disorders, including nonpsychotic major depression (e.g., Elkin et al., 1989), recurrent depression (Frank et al., 1990), bipolar mood disor-

3

der (Frank et al., 1999), bulimia nervosa (BN) (Agras et al., in press), and binge eating disorder (BED) (Wilfley et al., 1993; Wilfley, 1999). For specific strategies on how to adapt IPT across the range of psychiatric conditions, the reader is referred to Wilfley et al. (1998).

IPT has also been studied in various populations including the elderly (Reynolds et al., 1999), adolescents (Mufson et al., 1999), couples (Foley et al., 1989), and patients with comorbid medical conditions such as human immunodeficiency virus (Markowitz et al., 1998). In addition, a number of new research applications are currently under investigation for various disorders, including dysthymia (Markowitz, 1994), posttraumatic stress disorder (PTSD) (Krupnick, in press), social phobia (Lipsitz, Fyer, Markowitz, and Cherry, 1999), body dysmorphic disorder (Veale et al., 1996a, 1996b), chronic somatization (Scott and Ikkos, 1996; Stuart, 1999), borderline personality disorder (Angus and Gillies, 1994), and anorexia nervosa (McKenzie et al., 1999). Not surprisingly, IPT has been translated into several languages (for a review, see Weissman et al., 2000) and modified for group (Wilfley et al., 1993; Wilfley, 1999) as well as for long-term treatment (Frank, 1991).

THEORETICAL FRAMEWORK OF IPT

IPT's foundations lie partly in the work of Adolf Meyer (1957), who considered psychopathology a result of maladaptive adjustment to the social environment. Harry Stack Sullivan (1953) stands as the person who most clearly articulated the interpersonal paradigm and popularized the term *interpersonal* as a balance to the then-dominant intrapsychic approach. Sullivan taught that psychiatry involves the scientific study of people and the processes that go on among them, rather than the exclusive study of the mind or of society. He believed that the unit of clinical study is the patient's interpersonal relationships and that people cannot be understood in isolation from them. In his theory, Sullivan posited that people have "relatively enduring patterns of recurrent interpersonal situations"[1] that can either foster self-esteem or result in hopelessness, anxiety, and psychopathology.

Sullivan developed a comprehensive theory of the connections between psychiatric disorders and interpersonal relations for the developing child in the family and for the adult in the multiple transactions of life. The roles of major interest to interpersonal psychotherapy occur within the nuclear family (parent, child, sibling, spouse); the extended family; the friendship group; the work situation (supervisor, supervisee, peer); and the neighborhood or community. The interpersonal approach views the relationship between social roles and psychopathology from two perspectives: in terms of disturbances in social roles that act as antecedents for psychopathology, and in terms of mental illness that can produce impairments in the individual's capacity to perform social roles. IPT is also associated with the work of John Bowlby (1982), the originator of attachment theory, who acknowledged the influence of early attachment on subsequent interpersonal relationships and psychopathology. In sum, IPT is derived from a theory in which interpersonal function is recognized as a critical component of psychological adjustment and well-being.

CONCEPTS AND METHODS OF IPT

OVERVIEW OF IPT

IPT was initially formulated not as a novel therapy but as an attempt to represent the current practice of psychotherapy for depression (Weissman et al., 2000). It was developed in the 1970s and defined in a manual by Klerman and colleagues (1984) as a time-limited treatment for depression. IPT makes no assumptions about the causes of depression; however, it does assume that the development of clinical depression occurs in a social and interpersonal context and that the onset, response to treatment, and outcomes are influenced by the interpersonal relations that exist between the depressed patient and significant others. IPT moves through three defined phases, each of which is associated with specific strategies and tasks for the therapist and patient. Though similar to many other therapies at the level of techniques and stance, it is distinct at the level of strategies. Its well-defined treatment strategies are aimed at resolving problems within four interpersonal problem areas: (1) grief, (2) interpersonal role disputes, (3) role transitions, and (4) interpersonal deficits.

INTERPERSONAL CONCEPTUALIZATION OF DEPRESSION

Depression is conceptualized as having three component processes: (1) *symptom function,* the development of depressive affect and neurovegetative signs and symptoms (sleep and appetite disturbance, low energy, etc.), which are presumed to have both biological and psychological precipitants; (2) *social and interpersonal relations,* interactions in social roles with other persons derived from learning based on childhood experiences, concurrent social reinforcement, and personal mastery and competence; and (3) *personality and character problems,* enduring traits such as inhibited expression of anger or guilt, poor psychological communication with significant others, and difficulty with self-esteem. These traits determine a person's reactions to interpersonal experience. IPT intervenes in the first two of these three processes: symptom function and social and interpersonal relations. Because of its relatively brief duration and low level of psychotherapeutic intensity, IPT is expected to have little marked impact upon enduring aspects of personality structure, although personality functioning is assessed. On the other hand, many IPT patients gain new social skills that may help compensate for personality difficulties. An essential feature of IPT for depression is the intentional avoidance, during treatment of the acute symptomatic episode, of issues related to personality functioning and character pathology.

IPT Compared with Other Psychotherapies

IPT is not the only psychotherapeutic approach to treating depression. Both cognitive and behavioral approaches are similar to IPT in that they were developed specifically for depression, have been tested, and have been shown to be efficacious in randomized clinical trials. As specified by Frank (1973), the procedures and techniques of many schools of psychotherapy share common ground. Important common elements include attempts to help patients gain a sense of mastery, combat social isolation, restore a sense of social belonging, and find meaning in their lives. A major difference among the therapies is their conceptualization of the causes of the patient's problems as lying in the remote past, the immediate past, or the present. IPT, for one, addresses *current* interpersonal relationships, as shown in the following list of its core features:

1. IPT is time limited, not long term.
2. IPT is focused, not open ended.
3. IPT addresses current interpersonal relationships, not past ones.
4. IPT takes an interpersonal rather than intrapsychic approach.
5. IPT takes an interpersonal rather than cognitive/behavioral approach.
6. Personality is recognized, but it is not a focus.

Phases of IPT

The *initial phase*, usually the first one to four sessions, includes diagnostic evaluation and psychiatric history and sets the framework for the treatment. The therapist reviews symptoms, diagnoses the patient as depressed by standard criteria (American Psychiatric Association, 1994), and gives the patient the "sick role" (Parsons, 1951). The sick role may excuse the patient from overwhelming social obligations, but it requires the patient to work in treatment to recover full function. The psychiatric history, recorded during the initial session(s), includes an interpersonal inventory, a review of the patients' current social functioning and current close relationships, and a description of his or her patterns and mutual expectations. Changes in relationships proximal to the onset of symptoms are elucidated; examples may include the death of a loved one, children leaving home, worsening marital strife, or isolation from a confidant. This review provides a framework for understanding the social and interpersonal context of the onset and maintenance of depressive symptoms and defines the focus of treatment.

The therapist assesses the need for medication as part of treatment selection based on symptom severity, past history and response to treatment, and patient preference, and then educates the patient about depression by explicitly discussing the diagnosis, including the constellation of symptoms that define the diagnosis and what the patient might expect from treatment. Next, the therapist offers an interpersonal formulation, linking the depressive syndrome to the patient's interpersonal situation within the framework of one of the four interpersonal problem areas noted earlier: (1) grief, (2) interpersonal role disputes, (3) role transitions, or (4) interpersonal deficits. The depression is diagnosed within a medical model and explained to the patient. Symptom relief begins with helping the patient understand that the vague and uncomfortable symptoms are a part of a known syndrome—one that responds to various treatments and has a good prognosis. Having identified the major interpersonal problem area associated with the onset of the depression, the therapist makes an explicit treatment contract with the patient to work on this problem area. When this focus is agreed upon, the intermediate phase begins. (The initial phase of IPT-G is detailed in Chapters 3 and 4.)

During the *intermediate phase* of treatment, the therapist pursues strategies defined in the manual by Weissman et al. (2000), which are specific to the chosen interpersonal problem area. For grief, defined as complicated bereavement following the death of a loved one, the therapist facilitates mourning and gradually helps the patient to find new activities and relationships to compensate for the loss. Interpersonal role disputes are conflicts with a significant other: a spouse, another family member, a co-worker, or a close friend. The therapist helps the patient to explore the relationship, the nature of the dispute, and options to resolve it. Failing this, the therapist and patient, together, may conclude that the relationship has reached an impasse and that it should be ended. Role transition includes any change in life status—for example, the beginning or end of a relationship or career, a move, promotion, retirement, graduation, or diagnosis of medical illness. The patient is helped to deal with the change by recognizing positive and negative aspects of the new role that will be assumed, along with assets and liabilities of the old role. Finally, the problem area of interpersonal deficits defines the patient as significantly lacking in social skills, resulting in problems in initiating or sustaining relationships. The goal is to reduce the patient's social isolation by helping to enhance the quality of existing relationships and encouraging the formation of new relationships. It is important to note that the problem area may change during the course of treatment or that the patient may have several related problem areas and either work on more than one or select the most salient or mutable one. (The intermediate phase of IPT-G is detailed in Chapter 5.)

The *termination phase* is not unique to IPT inasmuch as feelings about termination are discussed, progress is reviewed, and the remaining work is outlined. As in other brief treatments, the arrangements for termination are explicit and followed closely. (The termination phase of IPT-G is detailed in Chapter 6. See also Weissman et al. 2000, for a comprehensive discussion of IPT with clinical examples.)

THERAPEUTIC STANCE OF IPT

Each model of psychotherapy can be characterized in part by the positioning of the therapist in terms of the nature of the relationship with the patient and the level of therapeutic activity. IPT is quite explicit regarding these features: (1) The therapist is a patient advocate, not neutral. (2) The therapeutic relationship is not interpreted as transference. (3) The therapeutic relationship is not a friendship. (4) The therapist is active, not passive. (5) The therapist maintains an intensive interpersonal focus.

TECHNIQUES

Although IPT is distinct at the level of strategies, it is similar to many other therapies at the level of techniques (Weissman et al., 2000). Some of its most frequently used techniques include exploratory techniques, encouragement of affect, clarification, and communication analysis; other techniques include use of the therapeutic relationship, behavior change techniques, and adjunctive techniques. (See Weissman et al., 2000, chapter 8, for a description of how these techniques are implemented in individual therapy, and Chapter 7 in this book for a description of how these techniques are applied in a group format.)

ADAPTING INTERPERSONAL PSYCHOTHERAPY TO GROUP[2]

RELEVANT ISSUES IN ADAPTING IPT FROM INDIVIDUAL TO GROUP[2]

IPT delivered in a group format directly addresses many patients' concern that they are the only ones with a disorder of this type and severity, facilitates the identification of problems common to many patients, and provides a cost-effective alternative to individual treatment. Given the number and different types of interpersonal interactions that can occur in a group setting, the interpersonal skills that are developed there may be more readily transferable to their outside social life than the relationship patterns that are addressed in a one-to-one setting such as individual therapy. Moreover, a group modality has therapeutic features not present in individual psychotherapy—for example, interpersonal learning and cohesiveness (Yalom, 1995). Obviously, groups in which membership is based on diagnostic similarity (e.g., depression, binge eating) offer a radically altered social environment for patients who have become isolated, withdrawn, or disconnected from others. Group participation alone, therefore, may help patients break patterns of social isolation and self-stigmatization that contribute to the maintenance of the disorder. This is not to imply, however, that delivering individual treatments in a group setting will capture the opportunities provided by group psychotherapy. In fact, interventions effective in individual psychotherapy (e.g., in-depth individual exploration) may lose some of their potency in a group context or, more significantly, may undermine the establishment of the group as a cohesive working unit. In making the transition from individual therapy to a group format, then, the therapist needs to consider how to maintain the integrity of important elements of the individual treatment (e.g., effective change processes, the focus on each individual's work, patient and therapist roles, specific techniques) while adapting them to the group context.

Wilfley and colleagues' (1998) interest in the process of adapting individual IPT to a group format emerged from the first author's initial efforts to adapt two individually based treatments, cognitive-behavior therapy (CBT) and interpersonal psychotherapy (IPT)—both originally developed for the treatment of major depressive disorder (MDD) (Beck, Rush, Shaw, and Emery, 1979; Klerman, Weissman, Rounsaville, and Chevron, 1984) and later modified for the treatment of bulimia nervosa (BN) (Fairburn et al., 1991)—to a group format (IPT-G) for the treatment of binge eating disorder (BED) (Wilfley et al., 1993). The initial group comparative psychotherapy trial for BED revealed quite promising findings at posttreatment (Wilfley et al., 1993), similar to results from individually based CBT and IPT treatments for bulimia nervosa (Fairburn et al., 1991). However, the maintenance of change findings at the six-month and one-year follow-ups were not as robust as that in Fairburn and colleagues' long-term follow-up data (1993). These differences in maintenance of change led Wilfley and

colleagues (1998) to consider whether they had mad
lation of CBT and IPT across disorders (from BN to
ties (individual to group). Thus, in their subseq
NIMH-funded comparative psychotherapy trial for I
colleagues (1998) worked diligently to refine their ac
and IPT across disorders and modalities. Analysis
data from their treatment trial reveals that the treatm
this second trial were significantly improved over t
(Wilfley, 1999)[3]. Therefore, it is clear that the refined a
itated a more successful translation of CBT and IPT across disorders
and modalities.

In the subsequent sections, we illustrate the relevant issues necessary to adapt individual IPT to a group format. Within each section,
we discuss the general considerations involved in making adaptations and describe the modifications made to the original treatment
protocol. Note, however, that many of the issues raised here apply to
any effort to adapt an empirically supported treatment for alternative uses.

PRESERVATION OF THE HYPOTHESIZED CHANGE PROCESSES

In adapting an individual treatment to an alternative modality, we
were concerned, above all, with how best to preserve the hypothe-
sized change processes of the manualized treatment while capitaliz-
ing on the unique features of the new milieu. Hence, one must first
identify those elements that presumably constitute the "active ingredients" of the treatment, then determine how the altered therapeutic
context will affect their delivery. A group modality, for example, possesses therapeutic features not present in individual psychotherapy.
Groups, such as ours, in which membership is based on diagnostic
similarity offer an immediate social corrective for patients who are
certain that they are the only ones who engage in a shame-producing
behavior. Thus, as noted, group participation by itself may help patients break patterns of social isolation and self-stigmatization. Yet it

is also possible that interventions effective in individual psychotherapy may lose some of their effectiveness in a group context or, more significantly, undermine the establishment of the group as a cohesive working unit.

MAINTAINING A FOCUS ON EACH INDIVIDUAL'S WORK

In comparison to other interpersonally oriented approaches, IPT employs strategies that are very specific and focused on patients' identified problem areas (Weismann et al. 2000). In adapting IPT to a group format, we realized that it was critical to retain this exclusive and strategic focus on individual patients' interpersonal problem areas and, at the same time, to avoid the trap of merely providing individual therapy in a group setting. The challenge, in short, was to identify ways to maintain an intensive focus on patients' interpersonal goals while creatively exploiting the unique therapeutic features of a group modality. Likewise, the chosen therapeutic stance had to be compatible with IPT, yet appropriate for a group milieu. We addressed these concerns by (1) scheduling individual meetings with patients, (2) conducting the interpersonal inventory prior to the first group meeting, (3) providing a thorough orientation to group therapy, (4) mailing weekly group summaries to group members, (5) developing a therapeutic stance based on an interactional group model, and (6) using our understanding of the stages of development in brief psychotherapy groups to inform our interventions.

Individual Meetings with Patients.   The goals of IPT are to reduce psychiatric symptoms and to improve the patient's current interpersonal functioning (Weismann et al. 2000). In individual IPT, these goals are addressed in weekly therapy sessions between the patient and the therapist. To compensate for the loss of sustained, exclusive weekly attention to each member's individual goals, we added three individual meetings to the twenty, ninety-minute sessions of group psychotherapy that constitute the core of IPT-G. We sequenced the meetings to correspond with critical time points in the three phases of IPT. The individual meetings between the patient and the therapist—or, rather, therapists (as co-therapy is best used for this approach)—occur at pretreatment (two hours), midtreatment (one hour), and posttreatment (one hour).

The Pregroup Individual Meeting.   The pretreatment meeting is crucial for facilitating a patient's individualized work in the first phase of IPT-G. In individual IPT, the first five sessions are devoted to a detailed examination of the patient's interpersonal history (i.e., the interpersonal inventory) and to the formulation of problem areas and goals that will guide the therapeutic work (Weismann et al. 2000). In these critical sessions, the patient is also oriented in a more general way to the work of psychotherapy and educated about the nature of his or her disorder and the means by which IPT is used to bring about a recovery.

Although it is possible to undertake individual preparation in the presence of other group members, such an approach would simply not be an efficient or therapeutically valuable use of group time. Translating IPT to a group modality thus requires the implementation of alternative strategies for identifying interpersonal problem areas and imparting the necessary patient education to orient each member to the work of group psychotherapy. Therefore, in the pretreatment meeting, the therapists focus on identifying interpersonal problem areas, establishing an explicit treatment contract to work on problem areas, and preparing patients for group treatment.

The interpersonal inventory and identification of problem areas are conducted as specified by Weissman et al. (2000). Note, however, that additional adjustments to the standard IPT protocol have been necessary because of the distinct differences between individual and group therapies. For example, moving from an individual to a group format has meant giving up the opportunity to focus each therapy hour exclusively on an individual patient's problem areas and goals. Therefore, alternative methods had to be developed to impress upon the patient that the interpersonal goals are the centerpiece of his or her work.

After identifying a patient's interpersonal problem(s) (i.e., interpersonal deficits, role disputes, role transitions, or grief), the therapists work collaboratively with the patient to formulate concrete prescriptions for change, along with the specific steps the patient will take to improve social relationships and patterns of relating. The goals of treatment are expressed in language that is as specific and personally meaningful to the patient as possible. In addition, each patient is given a written summary of his or her goals and told that these goals will guide the patient's work in the group. (See Chapter 3 for samples of patient goals.)

Another modification of the protocol involves adequately preparing patients for group treatment. Their individual goals are linked with the work of the group. Patients are encouraged to think of the group as an "interpersonal laboratory" where ties to others can develop, where naturally occurring "impasses" in the formation of intimate relationships can be examined in detail, and where patients can experiment with new approaches to handling interpersonal problems. Patients learn various social skills while participating in a group (e.g., interpersonal confrontation, honest communication, expression of feelings), and, indeed, the main goal of the group is to help them apply these skills to their outside social lives.

Finally, the therapists demonstrate "how" the group will work by treating this individual session like a "mini-group." For instance, as a patient's disturbed patterns of relating in his or her current social network are identified, the therapists begin to anticipate with the patient how these disturbed patterns are likely to emerge in the context of the therapy group. Specifically, a patient with interpersonal deficits may be told that when she describes distressing experiences, she uses language that is vague and intellectualized—a verbal style that may confuse listeners and contribute to feeling misunderstood. Following this type of "in-session observation," the therapists elicit the patient's reactions and explore what it is like to receive such feedback in the group. This technique is essential for helping patients understand how the group will work and how elements of their interpersonal style may contribute to their difficulties in relationships.

Linking information from in-session interpersonal behavior to out-of-session interpersonal behavior is an immediate and concrete way to enhance interpersonal learning (Dies, 1994). Thus, patients with interpersonal deficits are encouraged to develop relationships within the group (with therapists and group members) as a model for developing other relationships, and patients with interpersonal role disputes are encouraged to solicit feedback on how they communicate so they can learn how to resolve disputes with their significant others. In short, the group interaction itself can be used as a potent intervention for patients.

The Midtreatment Individual Meeting.   The midtreatment meeting is scheduled in the middle of the "work" stage (between sessions 10 and 11). This meeting provides an opportunity to conduct a detailed review of each patient's progress on his or her individual problems and to refine interpersonal goals. The therapists re-contract with patients during this meeting, as a means of outlining and emphasizing the work that remains, in- and outside of the group, prior to the conclusion of treatment.

The Posttreatment Individual Meeting.   The posttreatment meeting is scheduled within a week after the final group session. The therapists use this final individual meeting to develop an individualized plan for each patient's continued work on his or her interpersonal goals. Therapists review the group experience and relationships developed in the group in light of the changes the patient has made and plans to continue to make in outside relationships.

Group Summaries.   In contrast to individual treatment, where patients have the undivided attention of the therapist, in the early phases of group formation, patients may feel overlooked or confused about how others' interpersonal problems relate to their own. They may also feel disoriented by the sheer volume of information being imparted and by the emotional intensity of the group. Patients respond in a variety of ways to the anxiety of entering into group life: Some may seek to monopolize the group's time and attention; others may silently retreat into the background. Although IPT-G therapists are quick to intervene in ways that clarify and bring order to the unfolding process of the group, the ninety-minute period is invariably too brief a time to maintain both an intensive focus on each of the patient's interpersonal goals and an intensive focus on the development of the group as a therapeutic milieu.

To address this problem, group members are provided with weekly group summaries (a method adapted from Yalom, 1995) prepared by the group therapists following each session and mailed to group members at least twenty-four hours before the next session (the same set is mailed to all nine group members). These four- to five-page summaries focus on the transactions that occurred during each session and their implications for *each* patient's recovery. In particular, the notes help patients concentrate on making changes in problem areas in their outside social relationships. Each set of notes also includes information about the group process, the common interpersonal problems of those in the group (e.g., difficulty expressing feelings, excessive caretaking of others to the detriment of meeting their own needs, conflict avoidance), and how to use the group most effectively (e.g., how to use feedback and learn from other members' work on problem areas). The notes not only stimulate patient reflection between meetings and remind patients of their responsibilities to continue the work of the group in their outside social lives; they also appear to accelerate the pace of treatment. (See Chapter 8 for a sample copy of a group summary.)

THERAPEUTIC STANCE

In IPT, therapy involves identifying interpersonal problem areas and then using the therapeutic relationship to promote interpersonal development (Weismann et al. 2000). Well-established techniques such as clarification and encouragement of affect, improvement of communication skills, reassurance, and testing of perceptions and performance through interpersonal contact are the mainstays of treatment. These techniques have been incorporated fully into IPT-G.

However, a decision needed to be made about what therapeutic stance to take in relation to the group, in order to promote interpersonal development and to use the group to its maximum therapeutic advantage. Indeed, we realized that it was important to find a therapeutic stance flexible enough to incorporate the above-mentioned techniques into a semistructured group interpersonal learning environment. Approaches inconsistent with these aims—for example, Gestalt, Tavistock, and psychoanalytic—were rejected.

What we *did* find compatible with the overall goals of IPT is an interactive approach (Yalom, 1995) that emphasizes fostering direct communication between members. Such an approach also emphasizes establishing a safe environment where patients can receive feedback on how they are perceived by others and can experiment with new and risky interactional styles.

A unique feature of this interactional approach is the "in vivo" demonstration of characteristic problems in relating. The notion of "social microcosm" applies here. Skills that patients learn while participating in an interactive group setting (such as communicating clearly, tolerating interpersonal differences, and resolving conflicts with one another) can be applied to relationships in their outside lives. Also well suited to this approach is the IPT technique of communication analysis. For example, therapists can ask a patient struggling with a role dispute to recall (in great detail) a recent interaction or argument he or she had with a significant other. Difficulties in communication can then be identified and solutions to the problem interaction generated. Therapists can also ask group members if they have noticed similar problematic patterns between this patient and other members of the group—a question that often generates immediate feedback applicable to the patient's outside social life.

STAGES OF DEVELOPMENT IN
BRIEF PSYCHOTHERAPY GROUPS

As noted, IPT moves through three phases (i.e., initial, intermediate, and termination), each of which is associated with specific strategies and tasks for therapists and patients (Weissman et al. 2000). These phases are defined in such a way as to guide therapists in helping individuals identify problem areas, work on their goals, and consolidate their work in treatment. However, although the phases reflect an individual's progression in IPT-G, they do not reflect the stages of group development, nor do they provide intervention strategies for fostering healthy group development.

To remedy this problem, we used a stage-oriented group approach (MacKenzie, 1994a) to complement the structure and therapeutic tasks of the three phases of IPT (see Table 1.1). This model of group development parallels the developmental sequence of the three phases of IPT. The developmental sequence of a group emerges naturally, but successful movement from one stage to another can be disrupted by an ineffectual leadership style and by ill-informed intervention strategies (MacKenzie, 1994a). At best, therapists unaware of group development may use interventions that lead to an impasse (e.g., by allowing the group to become bogged down by "story telling"); and, at worst, they may use strategies detrimental to an individual's progress (e.g., by ignoring conflict to the point where it erupts and injures a patient). Therefore, in order to manage the group effectively and to develop a healthy group milieu, therapists need to understand the stages of group development (again, see Table 1.1).

Attending to these normative transitions in the group intensifies group cohesiveness, prevents premature dropouts, and assists patients in making otherwise difficult interpersonal transitions (MacKenzie, 1994a). Therapists who can predict critical transition points are able to create deliberate interventions to foster the work of the group. Thus, therapists use "stage-appropriate" intervention

TABLE 1.1 Linking the Phases of IPT to the Stages of Group Development

IPT Phases/Tasks	Group Stages	Members' Work	Therapist Interventions
Initial Sessions 1–5: Identify problem areas.	*Engagement* Sessions 1–2	Members look for structure as they grapple with the anxiety of being in a group and sharing their problems.	Therapist establishes a structure that encourages appropriate self-disclosure and facilitates norms for effective communication.
	Differentiation Sessions 3–5	Members work to manage negative feelings over inter- personal differences as these emerge in the group.	Therapist helps members understand their reactions in the context of inter- personal differences in their outside social lives.
Intermediate Sessions 6–15: Work on goals.	*Work* Sessions 6–15	Members work out differences and strive toward common goals.	Therapist facilitates connections among members as they share their work with each other and encourages practice of newly acquired social skills inside and outside the group.
Termination Sessions 16–20: Consolidate treatment.	*Termination* Sessions 16–20	Members struggle with how to manage the impending loss of con- nection with other group members.	Therapist helps members to consolidate their work and to plan continued work and assists members in grieving over the loss of the group.

strategies to help patients negotiate the developmental sequence of the group.

The stages of group development mirror the development of interpersonal relationships. For instance, involvement in the group requires that patients learn how to engage one another (in the *engagement* stage), how to cope with conflict and make rules for conflict management (in the *differentiation* stage), how to develop intimacy (in the *work* stage), and, finally, how to manage loss successfully (in the *termination* phase). Indeed, by helping our patients negotiate the stages of developing relationships within the group, we provide invaluable learning opportunities about how to work through the process of developing, sustaining, and ending meaningful relationships. (See Chapter 2 for further clarification of group stage development.)

Having provided the background of IPT and the relevant issues in adapting IPT for group, we can continue with our discussion of how to administer IPT-G. First, however, it should be noted that the majority of clinical case material presented in this book has been derived from the NIMH comparative psychotherapy study for binge eating disorder (the only empirical study of IPT-G to date) (Wilfley, 1999) and, therefore, much of this case material references the clinical and diagnostic features of BED. Nevertheless, given the comorbidity associated with BED (e.g., major depressive disorder, anxiety disorders, Axis II personality disorders), all of the case material presented will be relevant for clinicians and researchers who wish to use IPT-G with other diagnostic groups.

NOTES

1. Harry Stack Sullivan, *The Interpersonal Theory of Psychiatry* (New York: W. W. Norton, 1953), p.13.

2. The authors are indebted to Mary Ann Frank, Ph.D., Emily Spurrell, Ph.D., and Bruce Rounsaville, M.D., for their involvement in formulating the specific adaptations outlined in this last section.

3. In the Wilfley et al., 1999 large-scale (n=162) NIMH-funded comparative psychotherapy study for binge eating disorder (BED), IPT-G rivaled the effect of CBT in the short and long term across multiple domains. The effect sizes for both CBT and IPT are comparable to the best outcomes found with individual treatment.

CHAPTER 2

The Time-Limited Group
As a Treatment Modality

This book has been developed as a manual for applying the principles of IPT in a group format. It is not a comprehensive introduction to group psychotherapy, though many aspects of group management are described. It is assumed that clinicians using IPT-G will have clinical competency in conducting intensive psychotherapy groups. Some guidelines regarding such training are discussed in Chapter 9. We have tried to develop the manual in a way that is both comprehensive enough for use in formal empirical studies and comfortable for use by clinicians.

There have been several adaptations of IPT for conditions other than depression, as described in Chapter 1. These have primarily focused on considering how the standard principles of IPT can be applied to the specific symptoms found in the chosen patient population. Adapting IPT for use in groups has involved a different set of challenges—again, as described in Chapter 1. One such challenge is how to effectively use the group to maintain the intensive interpersonal focus found in individual IPT. This approach involves the development of a cohesive interactional group milieu that is then guided into consistent application of the IPT therapeutic strategies.

IPT and IPT-G are considered semistructured therapies because they prescribe as well as prohibit some aspects of technique. The result is a set of clear guidelines to keep the therapist "on model." This approach has proven to be effective for containing the diverse range of issues that group members bring to the group, while still addressing their goals effectively within a time limit. For experienced group psychotherapists, the principal task is to restrain themselves from using some of the techniques they have learned from other types of group psychotherapy. In applying this manual, the clinician is encouraged, first, to read the general description of conducting time-limited groups as presented in this chapter and, then, to read about the detailed IPT-G techniques and strategies in subsequent chapters for specific applications.

One important aspect of treatment manuals is to identify techniques and procedures that are unique to the model and those that are of a general nature—that is, to distinguish between specific and nonspecific features. This distinction is particularly important regarding the use of groups. The label *group psychotherapy* tends to be used generically, with the implication that a group is a group. But in actual practice, groups vary widely in terms of the therapeutic procedures employed. Most of the treatment manuals designed for use with the group modality have been concerned with highly structured psychoeducational or cognitive-behavioral models (McKay and Paleg, 1992). These models have tended to view the group in a *classroom* mode rather than an *interactional* mode. One of the advantages of using IPT in a group format is the natural alignment between the interpersonal focus of IPT and the interpersonal arena provided by a group. Chapters 3 to 6 delineate in detail how this can be accomplished.

Psychotherapy treatment manuals are also designed to specify unique techniques that allow discrimination between psychotherapy models. Such manuals have become essential for formal psychotherapy research and are increasingly being incorporated into clinical settings. They offer a number of potential benefits (Carrol and Nuro, 1997), which include the following:

1. Psychotherapy treatment manuals provide a means for objective comparisons of different psychotherapies.
2. They set standards for training and evaluation of therapists.
3. They establish clear treatment goals and clinical care standards.
4. They facilitate transfer of promising treatments from research to clinical settings.
5. They provide a means of linking treatment processes to outcome.
6. They reduce the variability in outcomes due to therapist effects.

Therapeutic activities can be classified into four categories of interventions, behaviors, or processes (Waltz et al. 1993): Those that are unique and essential, those that are essential but not unique, those that are acceptable but not essential, and those that are proscribed.

The first part of this chapter addresses the nonspecific aspects of time-limited group psychotherapy, particularly those that are essential but not unique. These are features that apply to all groups, although they may be emphasized to a greater or lesser degree. One might think of them as the essence of *groupness*.

The latter portion of this chapter and the relevant subsequent chapters address the aspects of IPT-G that are unique and essential.

EFFECTIVENESS OF GROUP PSYCHOTHERAPY

Group psychotherapy has occupied a significant portion of the psychotherapy landscape since World War II. Currently, there are increased pressures within the healthcare field to expand the use of groups. These pressures are easily discounted as being based primarily on financial concerns. Although it is true that the group format offers a more cost-effective means of delivering psychotherapy, there is also extensive empirical literature on the clinical effectiveness of groups. Group psychotherapy is not a second-rate treatment, nor is it limited to basic supportive functions. Several meta-analytic reviews indicate that formal psychotherapy provided through a group format produces the same outcome results as a similar type of psychotherapy in an individual format (Smith, Glass, and Miller, 1980; Shapiro and Shapiro, 1982; Tillitski, 1990; Piper and Joyce, 1996; McRoberts et al. 1998). This is true across a variety of diagnostic populations and treatment models. It is helpful for the group clinician to be able to cite this empirical background, because some patients may respond to the recommendation of a group approach with some concern. The pretherapy preparation procedures described in this manual (Chapter 3) are designed to address patient attitudes.

ESTABLISHING
THE GROUP FRAME

Effective psychotherapy is characterized by a carefully maintained frame (Gabbard, 1995)—a feature that is particularly relevant to group psychotherapy. The structure of the group experience needs to be carefully planned and executed in a way that allows the individual member to have a sense of basic security and predictability regarding what undoubtedly will be viewed as a potentially hazardous journey. Of course, organizing groups is a complicated, time-consuming process. Attention to detail during the initial stages will help to ensure that the group moves smoothly into its task. Pregroup activities include a clear definition of group goals and, therefore, of selection of members and preparation of members for the group experience. Modest structure in the early sessions promotes rapid cohesion (Kaul and Bednar, 1994). The importance of regular on-time attendance and guidelines regarding extragroup socialization must also be clearly emphasized.

GROUP COMPOSITION

Group psychotherapy has traditionally valued a heterogeneous member composition in order to provide a diverse range of interactional possibilities (Yalom, 1995). From this perspective, groups would be composed primarily on the basis of members' level of interactional capacity, taking into consideration such features as quality of interpersonal relationships, capacity to manage affect, and level of psychological mindedness. These groups could thus be termed homogenous in terms of capacity and heterogeneous in terms of symptoms and diagnosis. With the advent of various time-limited group models, however, the approach to composition has significantly shifted.

In principle, membership in time-limited groups is closed. All members begin and end together. In the service of clinical reality, however, it may be necessary to add members—over the first two or three sessions only. Any change in membership results in a need to reconfigure the relationship balance in the group and automatically sets back the level of group work. This can have a significant impact in time-limited groups. Longer-term groups are better able to adapt to a slow turnover of members. It is recommended that groups begin with seven to nine members. The loss of a member or two is not uncommon, and as membership drops below six, it becomes increasingly difficult to maintain a strong interactive group atmosphere.

In the time-limited literature, both individual and group applications fall within the range of twelve to twenty-four sessions.[1] The lower end of this range is commonly used for quite structured groups with a strong psychoeducational and skill development component. Groups take some time to become cohesive, a necessary process if the members are to engage in psychological work together. This objective requires the development of a basic sense of trust in the other group members. The group must be seen as a safe and supportive environment. Note that this entails an appreciation of the entire group system, above and beyond the individual members and the therapist. Twelve- to sixteen-session groups spend most of the first half becoming a truly working environment and most of the second half in the shadow of termination. For these reasons, groups of fewer than sixteen sessions tend to encounter constraints on the therapeutic possibilities involved and therefore need to be highly structured. Every session beyond sixteen increases the amount of working time and the opportunity for consolidation of gains.

Scheduling groups requires more detailed planning than scheduling individual psychotherapy. The dates of group sessions have to be carefully considered, taking into account holidays, long weekends, and so on. Since the number of sessions is limited, interruptions need to be as minimal as possible. As patients are assessed, the schedule should be reviewed in detail to ensure their availability at all sessions.

Given the double constraints of a time limit and the use of a group format, both of which make focusing tasks more difficult, homogeneous composition is essential. Homogeneous composition brings common target problems, thus enhancing motivation and facilitating the rapid emergence of a working focus for the group. This process, in turn, promotes early cohesion and an expedited movement through the crucial early stages of group development. It also creates an environment in which the members will feel almost immediately understood, often in contrast to their experiences in the outside world. For example, the members of a group composed of patients with treatment-resistant depression often report great relief that their struggles with the disorder are acknowledged (inasmuch as they are often unacknowledged by family and friends), and members of a binge eating group often experience relief at being able to talk about details of their eating behavior that they have kept a carefully guarded secret. This rapid sense of membership allows the group to get off to a fast start and, therefore, to have more time for advanced interactional work.

Specific caution is required regarding the presence of significant personality psychopathology among the members of a time-limited group. In particular, Axis II Cluster B symptoms of emotional lability and impulsivity will present serious challenges. Groups with a major loading of personality pathology require continuous attention to group process events in order to maintain the integrity of the therapeutic experience. Some members may terminate prematurely because they feel that a dominating member or a small subgroup has derailed their therapy.

In short, group composition requires system-level thinking. As a general rule, it is useful to identify patients who for some reason may not fit into the group or may cause significant problems for the group. Toward this end, we provide the following *member selection checklist*. Its guidelines should be considered not as absolute criteria but, rather, as elements of a screening guide intended to alert the group leader to possible difficulties. Only major discrepancies are relevant; minor fine-tuning of membership is not worth the effort.

As specified by this member selection checklist, exclusion is recommended in the case of an individual who

1. does not fully meet the purpose of the group (i.e., does not exhibit symptoms of binge eating disorder or major depression)
2. exhibits active suicidal ideation, or is involved in an acute and severe current stress situation
3. exhibits antisocial or psychopathic features
4. exhibits a highly defended personality style
5. possesses extremely low or no motivation to change

PRETHERAPY PREPARATION

The systematic preparation of patients for group participation has been shown to have positive effects (Kaul and Bednar, 1994), including enhancement of the rapid emergence of a cohesive group atmosphere and facilitation of the related goal of reducing early group dropouts. Almost everyone joining a group will have some apprehension, and a chance to discuss the proposed group in some detail is reassuring. The process of doing so also establishes a basic rapport between the therapist and the patient that helps to sustain members through the early sessions. Such a discussion is even more productive if the patient is given a handout about groups to read beforehand (see Appendix A). Another effective measure is open discussion about the duration of the group, including the date of the final session, as it gives the therapist an opportunity to respond to concerns or questions about the rationale for a time-limited approach. The importance of confidentiality should always be discussed since it will be a concern for almost everyone. And a brief mention concerning not coming to group under the influence of drugs or alcohol is useful to prepare for the management of such an event if it occurs. The goal is to create a tight and consistent experience that can make up in intensity what it lacks in time.

The management of contact with the therapist or with other therapists between group sessions should also be specified. As a general rule, in the service of keeping the playing field as uncluttered as possible, it is recommended in time-limited groups that individual sessions and other therapies outside of the prearranged frame of the group be discouraged. An exception to this rule would be less intensive contact for medication management. These guidelines should be accompanied by a general commitment that all contacts with professionals outside of the group will be discussed in the group by the member or, if necessary, by the therapist.

In time-limited groups it is not unusual for the therapist to contact a member who misses a session without notice; the same is true when indirect notice has been received. The goal of such contacts is to ensure that work on the target goals continues. This is an example of giving priority to the application of learning to outside circumstances more than to group process issues. Such therapist behavior might be frowned upon in a psychodynamic group where the nature of the group frame is more stringently defined.

Specific mention should also be made of attendance and punctuality. Missed sessions in time-limited groups have broader implications than those in individual therapy because of the deleterious effect on the entire group. In time-limited groups the number of sessions that can be missed should be specified. It should be made clear that the difficulty involved is related not to the individual reason for the absences but to the impact on group progress. In a sixteen-session group the absences should total no more than three, whereas a twenty-session group might allow a maximum of four absences. Stringency in this regard is based on the therapist's responsibility to the group. Erratic attendance may have a significant impact, in terms of continuity and cohesion, that interacts with the time limit to reduce the potential for a positive outcome for all members.

Socializing between members outside of the sessions also needs to be discussed. In groups where the interactional process is going to be significantly in focus, it is best to have a firm guideline specifying that such contact is discouraged. Bear in mind that patients often refer to therapy groups as "support groups," and that many may have participated in a group where socialization was promoted. Of course, groups by their very nature provide support, but it is wise to make clear, as members begin group, that they are now engaged in intensive psychotherapy and that becoming friends with other group members may make it difficult for them to use the group effectively. It is also useful to suggest that working on problems may cause them to feel more upset for a time as they address difficult and stressful issues.

Following is an overall *pretherapy preparation checklist:*

1. Discuss dates, time, and place of group. (A handout containing the schedule is recommended.)
2. Discuss attendance and punctuality, as well as the number of permissible missed sessions.
3. Discuss how to notify the therapist if unable to attend a session.
4. Discuss commitment to report unpredicted outside professional contacts.
5. Discuss commitment to report extragroup contacts.
6. Clarify the management of medications, if indicated.
7. Discuss the total number of sessions, and specify the date of the last session.
8. Provide information about the timing of a follow-up visit, if planned.
9. Provide a handout regarding information about group therapy: (a) myths about groups, (b) how to benefit most from the group experience, (c) confidentiality, (d) extragroup socialization guidelines, and (e) no alcohol/drugs.

PLANNING OF THERAPIST
ACTIVITY LEVEL

There are a variety of ways to approach group process structuring. These methods range from use of a detailed agenda to maintain control of process, to moderate control through group exercises, to structure through active focusing techniques, to relatively unstructured groups that have a general common direction or thematic focus. This spectrum is more or less associated with higher to lower levels of therapist activity (see Table 2.1). It is crucial for the therapist to have a clear sense of the type of structure to be employed and to be consistent in maintaining it. A constantly shifting structure would fragment the group and impede effective group development.

All time-limited group models emphasize the importance of the therapist being prepared to be active in the service of maintaining a focus on a range of predetermined areas of clinical relevance. Thus a change of role is required for clinicians who have been trained in longer-term models where the expectation is that issues will emerge over time and at a pace determined by the patient. Time-limited therapy turns this around completely. Issues to be addressed are determined at the beginning, and there is the pressure of the time limit to address these issues immediately and apply what is being discussed to outside circumstances at an early point. This circumstance requires clinician confidence and the incorporation of focused, yet supportive, techniques.

Semistructured groups make major use of the interpersonal elements of the group format. Facilitation around the interpersonal material will lead to more extensive disclosures regarding current relationships and possible linking to early relationship patterns. Although the emphasis is primarily on current relationships, identification of interpersonal patterns connected to earlier figures, especially in the family of origin, is expected. The inevitable result is greater affective intensity, which requires skillful management to utilize but contain the emotional component.

TABLE 2.1   Comparison of Time-Limited Group Models

Model	CBT	IPT-G Interpersonal	Yalom Interpersonal/ Interactional	Psychodynamic
Time frame	Time-limited	Time-limited	Time-limited, longer term	Time-limited longer term
Group schedule	Closed	Closed	Open/Closed	Open/Closed
Composition criteria	Common diagnosis or situation (e.g., binge eating, depression)	Common diagnosis or situation (e.g., binge eating, depression)	Common interactional capacity	Common interactional capacity
Formal pregroup preparation	Moderate: Incorporated into early sessions	High: Incorporated into early sessions	Low	Low
Therapist style	High activity	Moderate activity	Low/moderate activity	Low/moderate activity
Group structure	High: Programmed sessions	Moderate: Problem areas/goals established and actively kept in focus	Low/Moderate	Low/Moderate
Process focus	Low group process focus (managed to preserve teaching environment)	Moderate group process focus (managed to preserve group integrity, not interpreted)	High "here and now" group process focus (interpreted re interpersonal conflict)	High "here and now" group process focus (interpreted re intrapsychic conflict)
Homework	Written homework and behavior change expected	Changing interpersonal/ social patterns expected	Not formally prescribed	Not formally prescribed
Mediating strategies	Identify and block negative cognitions	Identify and alter current interpersonal/ social coping	Promote here-and-now interpersonal learning and existential awareness	Identify and understand interpersonal and intrapsychic conflicts
Focus on affect	Low/Moderate	Moderate (identification of excessive or blocked affect re current inter- personal tensions)	Moderate/High	Moderate/High
Extragroup socializing	Permitted, perhaps encouraged re assigned tasks	No	No	No

The imposition of structure is through strategic group management, and it is expected that much of the therapeutic potential will be delivered through the vehicle of group interaction via therapist activity level. In the first few sessions of the group, the therapist is quite active as he or she attends to the development of a cohesive working group environment. When positive group process norms are in place, greater attention can be devoted to the specific interpersonal issues of individual members. The therapist encourages active application of each member's work to outside relationships. The group is then used to review and discuss how these changes are being implemented and experienced. The role of specific intragroup interactions is not emphasized, and these will be managed more than explored.

USE OF CO-THERAPY

Co-therapy is a more complex model than solo therapy. It requires therapists who can work closely together in a collaborative manner. In time-limited groups, the cleaner the field of action the better. Poorly functioning co-therapists may introduce process difficulties into the group and be quite unaware of the results of their efforts. In more structured psychoeducational or skill-focused groups, there may be somewhat less need for concern. However, when the principal task of the group is to maintain an intense focus on interpersonal issues, the nature of co-therapy functioning may be critical to a successful outcome (Roller and Nelson, 1993). To date, there is no empirical evidence regarding the relative effectiveness of individual versus co-therapy models.[2]

It is useful to consider what conditions would justify the use of co-therapists and the accompanying doubling of staff resources. The worst possible rationale is therapist insecurity. If therapists are reluctant to lead a group alone, then they should not be conducting an intensive interpersonal psychotherapy group together. On the other hand, a well-functioning co-therapy pair can provide a complementary style of leadership that contributes to the effectiveness of the group. As treatment complexity and challenge increase, there may be an argument for co-therapy. For example, as the level of personality pathology becomes greater, there is higher pressure on the therapists to become enmeshed in unhelpful reciprocal patterns with the members. Such situations generally also contain a theme of splitting the therapists into idealized good and bad figures. Two therapists may be in a better position to identify such developments and deal with them. This is a task for experienced group therapists who are able to work together in close collaboration.

Co-therapy can also be a good training model, with clearly identified senior and junior roles that gradually merge in activity level as the group progresses. Another rationale for the use of co-therapists is to combat clinician burnout. In programs where clinicians lead a number of groups each week, the impact of the group atmosphere can become oppressive. To maintain vitality and provide peer support, the use of co-therapy in some of the groups may contribute to greater clinician commitment and enthusiasm—qualities important for sustaining a positive and cohesive working atmosphere.

Co-therapists should have a serious discussion about their style of group work. Although these need not necessarily be the same, they do have to be applied in a collaborative and integrated fashion. Often co-therapists divide their tasks to some extent, with one therapist focusing on the individual and the other considering the rest of the group. These roles may shift as different members come into prominence. It is wise to allow protected time for co-therapists to talk at least briefly before each session, and certainly at more length at the end of each. Such a pattern can be started with joint assessment of potential group members. An atmosphere of trust and openness is required for this procedure, along with a willingness to address the tensions that will inevitably arise between co-therapists.

The use of co-therapists provides an opportunity to model a constructive female-male relationship. For some patient populations this may be particularly relevant. For example, IPT-G groups have been developed for eating disorders, a population in which gender issues are often predominant and there is a substantial incidence of traumatic histories. A mixed-gender leadership would make good sense in such groups, whereas a male-male combination is probably contraindicated. The subtleties of the co-therapists' interactions require continual attention, since the modeling rationale often centers on roles that may be subject to gender biases that the therapists may be unaware of or unwilling to acknowledge.

It is easy for subtle competition to emerge between co-therapists, and to interfere with effective continuity. Patients are very aware of the nuances of the interaction between therapists, and the opportunity for splitting mechanisms is always present. The co-therapy relationship will reflect the same developmental phenomena as the group itself. So increased tension is predictable during the differentiation stage, when therapists may find themselves facing more disagreement about how best to intervene. (A growing disparity in activity level between therapists is perhaps a tell-tale warning sign.) For these reasons, co-therapists must have a strong commitment to reviewing their sessions together and an agreement that any source of tension between them is immediately open for discussion.

GROUP DEVELOPMENT

Group development has a lengthy empirical history, with reasonable agreement about the principal stages involved (MacKenzie, 1994a). The format of a time-limited closed group is ideal for tracking the environment of the whole group in terms of sequential phases. The therapist is in a position to reinforce phase-appropriate behaviors and thus to accelerate the group into a full working mode as early as possible. In the first few sessions, the group dynamics are used in the service of molding the group-as-a-whole more than dealing with specific members. Thus, the therapist must become competent in assessing the nature of the group process as a focus separate from the issues of individual members.

In a twenty-session group, for example, the first five sessions—the initial phase—would deal primarily with *engagement* tasks. The principal goals during this phase are to create a cohesive group atmosphere, establish positive group norms, and promote an active

member-to-member interactional atmosphere built around understanding the focal issues that each member has identified during assessment. The supportive group therapeutic factors of universality,
acceptance, and altruism drive the engagement tasks. These mechanisms are unique to the group setting; they are based on the interaction between the members, not on the therapist. The therapist's role
is to set the frame within which these mechanisms can operate, to
subtly reinforce their emergence, and to ensure that all members are
participating. The therapist is particularly active in maintaining the
focus of discussion on the identification and elaboration of the problem areas and target goals of each member. Thus, from the beginning,
the group forms around the critical issues that will need to be addressed. As this process of group formation proceeds, it is accompanied by a sense of hope that change is possible. This is a major
motivating force that is frequently accompanied by an early decrease
in symptom intensity. The therapist's central concern during this *engagement stage* is how the group is developing and how each member
is collaborating in this process. Information that is revealed about individual issues becomes, for the therapist, a source of connections between the members as they strive to clarify their issues in greater
detail.

Toward the end of the engagement stage, but prior to the beginning
of the intermediate phase of treatment, it is useful to consider a brief
interim stage termed the *differentiation or conflict stage* in the group literature. This stage is characterized by a challenging or critical tone on
the part of group members, along with a greater self-assertion that
contrasts with the largely positive atmosphere of the *engagement
stage*. Common themes include not getting enough advice or guidance, a desire to spend more time on earlier life events rather than on
current circumstances, and a resistance to accept that group psychotherapy is going to require serious applied personal work. This
stage provides an important impetus toward deepening group interaction. The development of an atmosphere in which personal issues
can be not only explored and supported, but also challenged, creates
a deeper capacity for effective work. It is important that therapists

appreciate this transition process and come to accept it as a positive sign of group development. Indeed, the principal task for the therapist is to encourage ventilation of issues and to refer them into the group for discussion. In this way they will be managed in the service of developing the group's capacity to deal with a broader range of challenges. Much of the task of interpersonal learning is enacted between members, not directly through the therapist. Thus, if tensions in the group are not addressed, there is the danger that a restricted atmosphere may prevail, shutting down the free flow of opinions and reactions that are essential to the interpersonal learning process.

The intermediate phase (sessions 6 to 15) of treatment—also called the *work stage*—is occupied with the central task of addressing each member's problem areas. The careful development of a strong working atmosphere in the initial sessions now pays off with a group capable of providing both support and challenge. It is expected that members will actively apply their group learning to their current life situation. The clarification of goals now shifts to the changes required to address them. The leader must encourage a sense of group enthusiasm for the work of each member and a curiosity about how external application is progressing for each. The members should drive the work of these middle sessions, a process that involves encouragement, support, and modeling on the part of the therapist, as well as confrontation and clarification of issues. Therapy is conducted through the group interactional process, and the therapist's role is to keep the group and its members on target.

The group leader must be alert to two common problems during the intermediate phase that may interfere with application to the patient's current psychosocial context. (1) As more is revealed about sensitive issues, the patient may tend to to dwell on past circumstances. The leader has a responsibility to keep the group in focus concerning the essential task of application to their lives now. This entails accepting past historical material with appropriate understanding, but taking the additional step of appreciating how past events influence current situations. Consideration might be given to an optional individual session at the midpoint of therapy to review interpersonal issues in more detail, so as to identify areas that have not received active attention.[3] Alternatively, this measure can be implemented by a group go-around in which each member's goals are discussed. (2) As the group interaction deepens, members may become absorbed in the group interaction for its own sake as a substitute social environment. Indeed, many people enter psychotherapy partly in order to address feelings of interpersonal dysfunction or social isolation. To feel understood and accepted may be a rare experience for them. The group may appear to be the solution, not the treatment, for what they need. The therapist must continuously address these two pressures in a constructive but firm manner.

The termination phase of the group encompasses the last five sessions. The therapist has the challenge of clearly identifying this transition point and the shift of focus it entails. Among group members there will be a sense of urgency in addressing work in progress that connects with the theme of now taking on personal responsibility for continuing application. Often new material will be introduced that needs to be confined so that termination can be addressed. Throughout the final sessions, then, it is helpful to encourage an exploration of the affect being experienced at the thought of ending. Identification of plans to maintain therapeutic gains and prepare for challenges is appropriate, as is identification of achievements. The final session provides an opportunity for clear statements of good-bye in an organized manner. Attention to the process of termination during these five sessions prepares the members to deal with the ending and promotes continued application of therapeutic strategies. An optional individual session immediately after the group terminates may be used to underscore changes made and goals for continued work.[4] A scheduled follow-up session serves as reinforcement for continued application and an opportunity to assess progress.

This basic schema of group development is helpful in that it keeps the therapist reminded of the trajectory of change and the shifting therapeutic emphasis as the group progresses. It also provides a template by which to assess whether the group is progressing "on schedule" with its work. (Recall that Table 1.1 in Chapter 1 compares the developmental aspects of IPT-G with the stages of group development.)

IPT-G IN COMPARISON TO
OTHER GROUP THERAPY MODELS

Group psychotherapy, like individual psychotherapy, may be conducted according to a range of possible theoretical models. All of these models provide the basic therapeutic mechanisms that develop from well-intentioned group interaction. These "common factors" are closely connected with basic interpersonal attachment processes that are in turn linked to core issues of self-esteem. A cohesive interacting group thus provides a powerful therapeutic atmosphere. The development of a sense of "groupness" is more complicated than the development of the therapeutic alliance in individual therapy. The guidelines in this manual for the initial phase of IPT-G are structured around the application of the supportive therapeutic factors that will promote early group cohesion.

Table 2.1 presents a comparison of time-limited group models. Note that groups based on cognitive-behavioral principles make use of the common issues related to a specific disorder or situation. In such cases the group is used for its motivational and amplification properties. The interpersonal group models are subdivided into the IPT-G and the Yalom models. Although both are focused on interpersonal issues, they differ in terms of process focus and mediating strategies. Psychodynamic groups share much in common with Yalom groups but make greater use of interpretive techniques.

In great detail, Weissman et al. (2000) discuss the various ways in which IPT differs from other individual psychotherapies. (This topic is also briefly reviewed in Chapter 1.) IPT-G shares those distinctions and is unique among group therapy models in other ways as well:

- *IPT-G is semistructured.* IPT-G is fully structured in terms of the manner in which the treatment is delivered (i.e., it offers distinct phases of treatment—namely, initial, intermediate, and termination—and it utilizes strategies for sharing interpersonal goals as well as strategies for working on designated interpersonal problem areas). However, it is less structured in terms of the manner in which each session is facilitated (i.e., it has no established agenda and no established thematic discussions, and it features an open interactive group milieu).

- *IPT-G is focused on outside interpersonal relationships.* IPT-G members are encouraged to keep their work focused on changing current interpersonal situations and/or intensifying important existing relationships. Although the group is used to manifest, alter, and examine important interpersonal situations and interactions, members are discouraged from using the group as a substitute social network. To limit this, the therapist discusses the matter with members at the pregroup meeting, and during the group itself, less emphasis is placed on intragroup processes and relationships unless they are specific to the work on a member's interpersonal problem area (e.g., interpersonal deficits).
- *IPT-G is action-oriented.* The IPT-G therapist places great emphasis on the transferring of interpersonal skills and insights learned in the group to the outside social network. The therapist also works actively in session to assist members in making relevant connections with one another around their interpersonal problem areas and goals. When appropriate, these in-session interactions are actively linked to relevant issues in the patient's outside relationships. A part of this process is the expectation that IPT-G members will work on their individual goals every day and come to the group prepared to talk about the changes they are making or attempting to make.

The four models summarized in Table 2.1 account for the great majority of clinical groups in use today. Each model is subdivided according to specialized techniques or target populations, but all have a common theoretical base. There is an active interest in the psychotherapy research community to establish more precise indications regarding the choice of group model for a particular patient or syndrome. It has been documented that the use of IPT with depressed individual patients results in better outcome when the techniques specified in the IPT manual are fully implemented (Frank et al. 1991). It is our hope that similar findings will emerge with further use of this IPT-G manual.

PRINCIPLES OF TIME-LIMITED GROUP PSYCHOTHERAPY

As a summary of this chapter, we now identify a few of the basic strategic principles of time-limited group psychotherapy. These principles form a structure around which the therapeutic process is organized. They also provide a yardstick for the therapist in gauging the progress of the group. When applied to an interpersonal group, their presence will be unobtrusive, and skillful application will make them seem logical and in harmony with the evolving atmosphere of the group.

1. Select an appropriate therapy model for the target population.
2. Assess patients for suitability with this model.
3. Prepare the patients for group and for the expectations of the model.
4. Set a clear time limit.
5. Compose the group in accordance with some aspect of homogeneity.
6. Ensure that all members fall into a generally similar range of interactional capacity.
7. Develop group cohesion around the areas of homogeneity and personal problem focus.
8. Promote an interactive group environment, and reinforce the supportive therapeutic factors.
9. Manage the discussion of group challenge to deepen the working capacity of the group.

10. Conduct a midpoint review of focus areas, and reinforce the time limit.
11. Deepen the focus on individual work in regard to affect expression and addressing problem areas and specific goals.
12. Expect and monitor outside application.
13. Focus on termination themes in the last five sessions.
14. Structure the final session with formal good-byes.
15. Schedule a follow-up individual appointment.

NOTES

1. In the NIMH comparative psychotherapy study for BED (Wilfley et al. 1999), a twenty-session format was used.

2. In the NIMH study (Wilfley et al. 1999), a co-therapy model was used. This was done for two reasons: (a) Given that the groups consisted of nine members each, it was thought that the addition of a co-therapist would be helpful in managing the group process while maintaining the interpersonal focus for all members. (b) The co-therapy format served as a training tool. Each IPT-G group was facilitated by a trained Ph.D. and an advanced graduate student co-therapist.

3. In the NIMH study (Wilfley et al. 1999), midtreatment individual sessions (between sessions 10 and 11) were held as a way to clarify the patient's interpersonal goals and to develop strategies for continued work in the group. See Chapter 1 for a more complete description of these sessions.

4. In the NIMH study (Wilfley et al. 1999), each patient was scheduled for a post-treatment meeting. These meetings were used to review the changes that came about as a result of treatment and to establish goals for continued work.

PART TWO
INDIVIDUAL ASSESSMENT
AND PREGROUP PREPARATION

CHAPTER 3

Assessment and Preparation for IPT-G

A GENERAL APPROACH TO ASSESSMENT

The assessment process has two principal goals: (1) to assess the patient adequately in order to make a diagnostic decision and decide on a preferred treatment course; and (2) to use the diagnostic information obtained to help the patient develop a reasonable focus for treatment. It is strongly recommended that such an assessment procedure be allocated a minimum of two interviews.[1] This is not an unreasonable time expectation for most service settings, especially in situations where the outcome is a decision to enter the patient into a treatment program that entails a significant expenditure of time, energy, and expense.

The patient is assessed in a standard diagnostic interview lasting approximately one hour. Through this interview, a DSM-IV diagnosis is established along with a general formulation that pulls together past development, current stress, and relevant psychological issues. The interviewer must therefore be selective in obtaining information related primarily to the diagnostic task. On the basis of this interview, a decision is made as to whether or not the patient is suitable for the group being planned. The possible use of medications is also a consideration, since IPT-G is designed for an integrated approach. In addition, a decision should be reached regarding the principal problem area to be addressed. The patient is given a written handout about group therapy (as discussed in Chapter 2) and may be asked to complete a set of investigator-based questionnaires appropriate to the specific program to be entered. The latter is encouraged, as the process of answering questions is helpful in preparing the patient for treatment. The assessment process can also be very therapeutic. For some patients it may be the first time they've had the opportunity to disclose the intimate details of their disorder to individuals with expertise in treating that disorder. It also stimulates an introspective process and helps to identify important issues that can be realistically addressed in the proposed treatment. Table 3.1 identifies some of the commonly used measures for use with individuals who struggle with depression or eating disorders. A brief description of each of these measures is contained in Appendix B.

In the second meeting, which also lasts approximately one hour, the principal task is to develop several target goals that serve to fine-tune the general strategies related to the problem area(s) to be addressed in treatment. In addition, the patient is educated about the group therapy and his or her role as a member.

It should be noted that the potential use of IPT-G for different diagnostic categories is yet to be fully tested. What we do know, however, is that IPT-G is not designed for use with severely dysfunctional patients. Several contraindications to recommending IPT-G as a primary or adjunctive treatment have been identified:

1. current drug or alcohol dependence
2. acute active suicidal threat
3. unwillingness and/or inability to establish a collaborative effort with the therapist
4. acute psychosis

TABLE 3.1   Commonly Used Assessment Questionnaires

For Completion by the Patient:

Category	Questionnaires
Symptoms	Symptom Checklist (SCL-90-R) Brief Symptom Inventory Outcome Questionnaire Beck Depression Inventory Emotional Eating Scale Eating Disorder Examination—Questionnaire
Interpersonal functioning	Inventory of Interpersonal Problems Structural Analysis of Social Behavior (SASB)
Social functioning	Social Adjustment Scale UCLA Loneliness Scale—Revised
Personality traits	NEO Personality Inventory (NEO-PI)

For completion by Clinician	
Global assessment	Global Assessment of Functioning (GAFS)
Investigator-based interviews	SCID (I and II) Eating Disorder Examination

THE INDIVIDUAL
PREGROUP MEETING

It is recommended that assessment and orientation tasks be conducted over a minimum of two sessions and a maximum of four sessions. More than four individual sessions make it increasingly difficult for the patient to give up the therapist for the unknowns of the group environment and are often not possible within managed care restrictions. During these meetings the therapist should keep in mind the following overall objectives:

1. Review the patient's current symptoms.
2. Establish a diagnosis and discuss it with the patient. (This discussion should include assignment of the "sick role."
3. Complete the interpersonal inventory.

4. Collaboratively establish the relevant problem area(s).
5. With input from the patient, develop a set of interpersonal goals that relate to the problem area(s).
6. Prepare the patient for the group experience by discussing the nature of work in the group.

The pregroup meetings are crucial for facilitating each patient's individualized work in the initial phase of IPT-G. Careful preparation will lead to a rapid and smooth beginning of the group. In individual IPT, the first five sessions are devoted to a detailed examination of the patient's interpersonal history (i.e., an interpersonal inventory) as well as to the formulation of problem areas and target goals that will guide the therapeutic work. In these critical sessions, the patient is also oriented in a more general way to the work of psychotherapy and educated about the nature of his or her disorder and the means by which IPT-G is used to bring about a recovery.

Although it is possible to undertake such individual preparation in the presence of other group members, this approach would not be an efficient use of valuable group time. Translating IPT to the group modality therefore requires the implementation of alternative strategies for identifying interpersonal problem areas, developing target goals, and orienting the patient to the group format. The individual pregroup meetings also allow the development of a working alliance with the patient that will be a sustaining supportive force in the early sessions of the group.

BEGINNING THE INDIVIDUAL PREGROUP MEETINGS

The pregroup meetings begin with a review of the recent history of the disorder and a review of the symptoms. The history of the disorder should include a review of past episodes—in particular, a search for interpersonal precipitants and/or consequences of the disorder and a discussion of the ways in which previous episodes were resolved. One useful method of streamlining and/or supplementing the review is to create a timeline table in which the patient lists relevant interpersonal events and their relationship to the disorder. An example is shown in Table 3.2.

Educating the patient about his or her disorder, including reassurance and guidance in managing symptoms, should be part of the pregroup meetings, because it establishes the patient's commitment to the treatment and creates a sense that the problems are being "worked on" right away. A "fact sheet" that provides information about the disorder and the rationale for treatment can also be helpful toward this end. (See Appendix C for an example of a fact sheet used in the NIMH study on binge eating disorder.) Initially, it is useful for the therapist to provide an overview of these meetings and to establish the goals to be met during the group sessions. IPT-G emphasizes the importance of maintaining a focus on goals, and the pregroup meetings provide a model of this approach. The following is an example of how a therapist might proceed after establishing a diagnosis of a woman who has binge eating disorder:

THERAPIST: It would be helpful to review a recent episode of overeating and talk about how that gets started and what exactly happens. And then we can go back to the time when you first were aware that you began to use food in that way. I know that you identified at least initially that you started binge eating at around age sixteen, so we will need to go back to your high school years and talk about what was going on then. After that we'll fill in the in-between years. One goal of this meeting is to right away begin to make connections between your binge eating and the way in which you have coped or managed with difficult interpersonal situations.

It is also useful during the pregroup meetings to talk repeatedly about the nature of the interpersonal treatment. These discussions

TABLE 3.2 Example of a Personal History Timeline Table*

Age	Problems	Relationships	Events/Circumstances	Moods
5	Normal weight		Tonsils are removed	
6	Begins gaining weight			
14			Grandfather dies	Feels sad at funeral but does not cry because she thinks it would be a sign of weakness
15	Concerns about weight; first binge; prescribed amphetamines to lose weight		Sister gets married, borrows money from parents, and files for bankruptcy with her husband	Perceives parents as being extremely disappointed in sister
16	Less concern about weight because "boyfriend's ex-wife was a lot heavier than me" but began binge eating	Meets boyfriend [Paul], 23, who works at a gas station	Does not tell parents about boyfriend, given father's high-profile job and position in the community	Comfortable in relationship; fearful of parents' disappointment; worries about their finding out
18	Binge eating when alone	Becomes engaged	Graduates from high school; goes to technical school	
		Tells sister, not parents	Abortion	
	Loses weight	Paul breaks off the engagement	Boyfriend "steals" back the ring (seen on his new girlfriend); throws herself into work as a secretary; is promoted repeatedly	
	More comfortable about weight ("boyfriend's wife was a lot heavier than me")	Meets new boyfriend, who works as a salesman; he says he is separated from his wife who is pregnant	Boyfriend's wife pickets her parents' house; parents do not make mention of this	Does not feel guilty about the relationship

TABLE 3.2 (Continued)

Age	Problems	Relationships	Events/Circumstances	Moods
	Binge eating when alone ("food was my only friend when he was away"); never ate when with him	Lies to family and friends, telling them that they got married	Moves to Minnesota with [new] boyfriend	Secrecy (wanting to be "perfect and not disappoint my parents"); homesick
		Spouse of co-worker tells her he is cheating on her	Throws boyfriend out of the house; on his way out he takes her ring from her jewelry box	
27	Binge eating as an outlet	Gets pregnant, marries the father [Bob], an alcoholic, who is "cruel and verbally abusive"	Lies to mother that she got pregnant after the wedding; birth of first child	Compliant, scared
28		Bob occasionally shoves her		Hateful
32	"Eating a lot"	Bob hits her; she stands up to him only once, to ask him to choose between her and alcohol	"I channeled my energy into my son"	Scared
		Bob no longer drinks but continues being verbally abusive	Does not tell anyone ("Nobody had a clue that we didn't have a wonderful marriage")	Emotionally distant ("I made it happy for me")
39		Has sex with husband approximately 2 times a year	Continues Den Mother activities; very active in church	Fearful that husband will hit her; obedient; proud at holding onto her feelings; derives esteem from keeping her trouble from her children and others
			Husband invests $20,000 of their joint money in real estate—all money lost; patient begins saving "every penny," sending $5,000 to her sister to open a savings account; became a workaholic	
41	Eating as a way to "hold everything together"	Sexual relationship with husband ends; although she does not express anger, he yells at her, saying he can do whatever he wants with his money		

(Continues)

TABLE 3.2 *(Continues)*

Age	Problems	Relationships	Events/Circumstances	Moods
46	260 lbs., highest weight ever; blood pressure increasing with increasing weight		Marital therapy with clergy for 3 months	
47	Loses up to 170 lbs.; lowest adult weight	Patient files for divorce		
50		Meets current boyfriend	Mother dies	
51		Moves in with current boyfriend		Funeral is "a lot less stressful [than my grandfather's] because I knew it was OK to cry"
52	Binge eating at night on objectively large amounts of food at least 3 times per week	Does not tell family members she is seeking psychological help	Works 14-plus-hour days, not pausing to eat or rest during the day2	Feels satisfied with their relationship
	Begins group psychotherapy			

*Table format adapted from Fairburn, 1998.

will provide patients with an understanding of how an interpersonal approach can be helpful, as there may be times when they have a difficult time making the connection between their disorder and the disturbances in interpersonal relationships that they have experienced. The following is an excerpt from a pregroup meeting in which the patient is initially unsure about whether interpersonal treatment fits her understanding of her binge eating:

THERAPIST: I was curious to get a sense about what makes taking a cognitive-behavioral approach to treatment seem like it made more sense to you in terms of a good fit?

BARB: I don't know. I just felt like the, it just fit as opposed to the interpersonal. That was the only reason. Interpersonal to me is, I don't think I have a problem with it, but maybe I do.

THERAPIST: And so when you think of that, when you say that you don't have a problem with your relationships you mean . . . ?

BARB: I have, you know, I have wonderful relationships and I have billions of friends. And that's not one of my problems. I'm an extrovert.

THERAPIST: I'll tell you a little bit about what interpersonal treatment is, and especially the importance of close intimate relationships, not just general socializing. One of the things that we're aware of is that people struggling with this problem of binge eating may have a difficult time managing stress, especially feeling that they are not able to set limits for themselves, you know, sometimes people may be real people-pleasers or work . . .

BARB: That's right.

THERAPIST: . . . work at taking care of other people and then consequently don't take care of yourself. And so then food becomes a way to manage the residual feelings or resentment that builds when you overextend yourself.

BARB: True, what you were saying is all me.

THERAPIST: And so in many respects if we look at it from that vantage point, we can also help you get your binge eating under control.

BARB: That's why I'm here. I want to get it under control.

GIVING THE SYMPTOMS A NAME

After the review of symptoms it is important to say that these multiple symptoms have a single clear name. Patients should be told that the syndrome of either their depression or their binge eating has been diagnosed, and that the symptoms they are experiencing are all part of the disorder.

In cases of depression, this point can be conveyed to the patient in words such as these:

THERAPIST: We've talked about these down periods you have and how they make it difficult to continue at work, and how you sometimes get so low that even living sounds impossible and that you find yourself wondering if it's even worth being alive. You have been experiencing episodes of major depression. Your symptoms of trouble sleeping, no appetite or energy, even trouble concentrating, and feeling irritable and on edge so you avoid your friends, all of these are typical of depression.

SUSAN: You know, my friends have told me that, but I just couldn't believe it, depression always sounds like a weakness or something, just being lazy.

THERAPIST: We know that a lot of people experience depression and that it can be effectively treated. One aspect of understanding your depression is to try to identify situations or events that might have occurred around the time of the episode.

SUSAN: But I thought depression was all about brain things, circuits and stuff.

THERAPIST: Well, there are some chemical changes that are associated with depression, but such symptoms are also often associated with a disruption of interpersonal relationships. That's one reason why a treatment approach like this one that focuses on interpersonal issues seems to be very helpful in treating depression.

SUSAN: You know, I guess I've had a hunch that I needed to look at that area but I never quite got the nerve up to do something about it.

For an eating disorder the description may sound like this:

THERAPIST: From the interviews we've done so far we're aware that you have a diagnosable eating disorder. It's called binge eating disorder. It's similar in many respects to some of the other eating disorders in that you have episodes where you eat a large amount of food, at times just feeling once you get started you can't stop. It's like a switch gets flipped and you almost move into automatic pilot and find yourself just eating.

BARB: That's the kind of control I don't . . . but I have great control in everything else that I do.

THERAPIST: That's right. Many people say that, their life is in pretty good shape and with everything under control except for this one area; like the eating disorder has taken on a life of its own.

BARB: I didn't know that it was a disorder.

GIVING THE PATIENT THE "SICK ROLE" AND RESPONSIBILITY IN ADDRESSING IT

The symptom review, the diagnosis, and the description of what the patient may expect, including the type and course of treatment, all serve deliberately to give the patient the "sick role." This role allows patients to receive in a compensatory but time-limited way the care that has not been adequately received, or felt as received, from others.

Describing the recovery process is helpful, because it limits the sick role and informs the patient of the obligation to cooperate in getting well and relinquishing that role as soon as possible (Suchman, 1965a, 1965b). The recovery phase should begin almost as soon as the patient is engaged in treatment.

A patient with depression might be introduced to therapy as follows:

THERAPIST: Addressing your depression is going to take some hard work. So part of your job will be to use the group to understand more about what goes on at those times. Do you have some ideas about where to start?

SUSAN: When I filled out that sheet on when I had depressions, it really got me thinking about how they all seemed to turn around me and guys. I feel sort of ashamed to talk about it, but I think I just seem to go all soft and passive-like when I get too close. I don't like that and it's not at all how I am at work. In fact, I know some of my boyfriends didn't like it either. So I guess I need to think about what that's all about.

THERAPIST: That sounds like an important part of the pattern. The group will be a useful to place to talk about that. You mentioned that you feel ashamed about it, so you will need to get up your courage and let the group know at an early point that this is something you need to address.

SUSAN: That's going to be hard. I think I learned a long time ago that it's not right to complain or feel sorry for myself and I can just hear my father saying "No more whining."

THERAPIST: It's good you mention that because sometimes these patterns do go back a long ways. So trying out a more assertive style in the group, and making sure you get your share of the action, would be important. It might be helpful to discuss how early experiences were important, but the real work needs to be on how you can make changes now both in the group and in your present relationship to see if the tension can be resolved.

The therapist might establish the sick role for a binge eating patient by saying the following:

THERAPIST: With the interpersonal treatment, the way that we think it's going to work and the reason why we think it's going to be helpful is the way you described situations where you overextend yourself, take care of others, and not take care of yourself. The natural course of that is just to end up feeling resentful or like nobody's taking care of you. Here you're putting out everything and nothing's coming back in. And oftentimes then food is to get what you're not getting from other people.

BARB: I've always said that food was my friend.

THERAPIST: And in many respects you're right, it's probably the one consistent thing that's been in your life that you have control over, that's always there, and it's always available. But if we can help move in a direction where you can begin to find ways to take better care of yourself, find ways to have relationships that are more equal, not that they're not good but to make them more balanced so you don't feel like you're putting out all the time, then you can make changes in the way that you're using food and get the binge eating to stop.

BARB: That makes sense. Yeah, it makes sense.

ESTABLISHING THE PROBLEM AREA(S)

As the therapist guides the patient through the review, the primary interest is in determining which interpersonal issues are most central to the patient's current eating disorder or depression and which aspects of the patient's difficulties are open to change. The therapist should obtain enough information to define the primary problem area(s). This is important because each problem area has a specified treatment strategy. Since IPT-G is a time-limited model, it is usually concentrated on one or two of the four problem areas. This classification of problem areas conceptualizes interpersonal problems according to a system that focuses on potential areas of change in treatment. The classifications are not exhaustive; they do not represent in-depth formulations, nor do they attempt to explain the dynamics of the disorder. Instead, this classification system is intended to help the therapist outline realistic goals and follow appropriate general treatment strategies.

In the following sections, each of the four problems areas is discussed in turn.

Grief.   It is common for depressive symptoms to emerge following the loss of a loved one and to last for up to a year after the death. However, some individuals suffer from prolonged grief reactions in which dysphoric symptoms do not remit, whereas others, who are seemingly functioning well, may exhibit hidden or distorted grief reactions that they have not consciously linked to the loss. Symptoms may begin or become exacerbated in the context of prolonged or distorted grief reactions, in which the painful feelings associated with the loss have not been addressed. A careful review of important life events can be helpful in recognizing the role of grief in the patient's behavior. It is common for patients with unresolved grief issues to experience a sense of feeling numb and cut off from life; they also may not remember feeling sad or upset. The therapeutic aim is to help these patients go through an open mourning process and then to find ways of filling the space left by the loss and becoming reinvolved in socialization. A key premise related to pathological grief is that the patient has not been able to grieve because of a fear of being unable to tolerate the painful affect associated with the loss. A supportive group provides an ideal environment in which to address grief work.

Interpersonal Role Disputes.   An interpersonal role dispute is identified when the patient and at least one significant other have nonreciprocal expectations about the roles that they should play in the relationship. The goal of treatment is to help the patient clearly identify the dispute and to begin to resolve it. This process entails an initial assessment as to whether the dispute is at a stage where active *renegotiation* of the relationship is possible. If not, the dispute may be at an impasse that, in itself, has a prolonged history and no effective resolution. The initial therapeutic task in such a situation is to strive to move the dispute into a stage where active renegotiation can occur. On the other hand, if the relationship appears to be essentially over and the desire for renegotiation is absent, then support for the patient to address *dissolution* may be in order. The group provides a context in which the patient can discuss and come to understand the dispute while also developing ways to manage and resolve disagreements. It also provides an opportunity to address interpersonal features that have been replicated in several relationships and, perhaps, identified in the group itself.

Role Transitions.   Symptoms may emerge in the context of adapting to a new set of circumstances, affecting patients at any point from late adolescence through old age. Both depressives and binge eaters may be well into middle age when they present for treatment. At this time of life they may be experiencing role-transition stress related to becoming a parent's caretaker, experiencing a job change or loss, making retirement plans, or losing a spouse. Since managing a role transition may involve the fear of losing one's sense of self-identity, the therapeutic goal is to help the patient get through the transition issues involved and thereby achieve a sense of mastery over the new situation. This process involves strategies similar to those used in addressing grief.

Interpersonal Deficits.   Interpersonal deficits are defined as profound and persistent disturbances in social relationships. Many of these difficulties are long-standing and have led to a failure to develop intimate adult relationships. Individuals with interpersonal deficits often lack social skills and have pervasive, maladaptive ways of reacting to relationships that prevent their social and emotional development. Such patients are often quite socially isolated or involved with others in such a superficial manner that the relationships are chronically unfulfilling. Their relationships are typified by a lack of emotional expression, avoidance of conflict, fears of rejection, and a lack of perceived support. The therapeutic strategy is to help these patients focus on the appropriate interpersonal difficulties and devise more successful strategies for handling them, thereby reducing their social isolation. In the process, the therapist can review the patients' past relationships with the aim of helping to discover the social behaviors that have led to failures. The group is an ideal setting for identifying "in vivo" the social difficulties with which patients are struggling and determining ways to improve social skills in the context of a therapeutic social milieu.

Patients may present for treatment with problems in more than one area. In such cases, an attempt must be made to establish a primary problem area that can serve as the initial principal focus. For patients with wide-ranging problems, the therapist may be guided in the choice of focus by the precipitating events of the current episode. Occasionally, however, the patient and the therapist may disagree about the appropriate focus. Some patients are unable or unwilling to recognize or acknowledge the degree to which a particular problem is distressing them. For example, patients with marital-role disputes may be reluctant to discuss these problems for fear of endangering the marital relationship. And patients with grief reactions may be unaware of the source of annual episodes of depression. Persistence in working with such patients to arrive at a mutually acceptable problem area will be rewarded as therapy begins.

DEVELOPING INTERPERSONAL TARGET GOALS

During the assessment process the therapist will be developing an understanding of the patient's past interpersonal functioning (e.g., family, school, social life); the patient's current interpersonal functioning (e.g., family, work, social life); the interpersonal precipitants of episodes of depression or binge eating; and the history of recent changes in all three. From this information, target goals will be developed, probably not more than three. To the extent possible, target goals should include reference to specific persons, specific events, and specific interpersonal themes. This helps to ensure that the target goals are expressed in language that is as specific and personally meaningful to the patient as possible. Following identification of a goal, the therapist will want to match concrete ideas for change, collaboratively identifying the specific steps that the patient will take to improve relationships and socialization. At an early point, each patient can be given a written summary of their goals that will provide a guide for work in the group. The final version of these goals will evolve over the early sessions.

It is useful to begin with a detailed description of the current episode and the surrounding interpersonal and social issues. Using this description as an anchor, the therapist can encourage patients not only to recall the first occurrence of episodes like the one they just described but also to recognize recurring patterns. The interpersonal inventory should be viewed as a tool for making ongoing connections between interpersonal themes and events on the one hand and symptomatic episodes on the other. It should include a focus on behaviors, cognitions, and affects. Throughout the interview the therapist should continually check with the patients to see how they are feeling when talking directly about sensitive interpersonal issues. In this way the therapist can provide practice in attending to and identifying current emotional states related to interpersonal stress that may trigger an increase in symptoms.

As a way of examining the interpersonal inventory process in detail, consider the following case example of an interpersonal inventory conducted with a woman with binge eating disorder. The primary problem area for this case is interpersonal deficits. As it is somewhat more challenging than the other three problem areas, it requires a thoughtful therapeutic approach toward establishing goals that are both attainable and meaningful over the course of a brief treatment like IPT-G.

REVIEWING A CURRENT
EPISODE OF THE DISORDER

THERAPIST: So give me a recent episode that . . . one of those when you felt like you just ate uncontrollably and couldn't stop yourself and had that bad feeling associated with it.

BARB: It must have been Monday night, I worked really late, until 8:30. Then I went to Taco Bell, and I hadn't eaten really all day. I must be the busiest clerk, I worked thirteen and a half hours without stopping. I probably drank like two big quarts of water, you know, big bottles of water.

THERAPIST: You're busy from morning until night when you work.

BARB: And I never stop, I never even take a lunch break. But Saturday and Sunday I don't have problems with my eating because my boyfriend's with me. I never ever have a problem when I'm around him. I ordered three things that I like and I ate two of those things before I ever got home, and then I just ate the last thing in the TV room with my boyfriend like it was the only thing I ordered. I was actually totally out of control.

THERAPIST: I appreciate you willingness to talk about that—it was a good example. One thing that I am immediately aware of is that you're not taking very good care of yourself.

BARB: (whispering) Oh, I know that.

THERAPIST: In terms of just those kind of hours . . . you're overextending yourself.

BARB: And you know, I am overextending myself. However, which customers am I going to tell I'm not going to be there? I can't say to people I'm only going to work from eight to five, because my clients all work. And I even get panicked if I think I have a two-hour hole in my day, I've got to fill that in, I've got to call somebody to see if they can come in.

The therapist's goal during the interpersonal inventory is to pay attention to the full range of issues that may currently be affecting the syndrome. In the above example, the therapist chose to focus on the patient's need to overextend herself. It is not unusual during this pregroup meeting for issues to emerge that may at first seem unrelated to the problem area. However, it is common during the exploration of interpersonal issues for patients to raise important issues that are in fact critical to a better understanding of the problem area. In this next section, notice how the discussion about taking care of self leads Barb to a discussion about her relationship with her ex-husband. As the interview continues into a review of the patient's past interpersonal relationships, the therapist keeps this information in mind (overextending self, working to hide feelings, maintaining a happy exterior) and begins to think not only about the relevant problem area but also about possible goals for treatment.

THERAPIST: Is your work schedule designed to keep things together financially, is it . . .

BARB: I was married for twenty-two years to a man I detested, and I'm trying to think . . . (crying)

THERAPIST: That's all right.

BARB: (crying) And I hated him but I stayed with him twenty-two years because I swore I would because of my son. And my son had no clue, I mean he had no clue. For twenty years I fooled everybody, everybody. I mean twenty years. And even my parents, nobody knew. I don't think he even knew, to tell you the truth, I don't think he even knew I was miserable. And he was cruel. He says that was not cruel, it was a joke. It wasn't. He was cruel about my weight.

After a review of a current episode, the therapist needs to turn the focus to the range of interpersonal issues that may be associated with the onset or maintenance of the disorder. During this discussion, the therapist works to understand what interpersonal events or episodes are associated with the disorder and, with the patient's input, begins to draw connections among these events.

REVIEWING PAST INTERPERSONAL FUNCTIONING

Therapist: Now, let's go back to when you first were aware that you were having eating episodes like you just described. I want you to think back and tell me what was happening in your life in terms of relationships, connections with other people, anything like that where you think that food had become a kind of friend.

BARB: I don't really think I binged, my mother made huge meals and we took our lunch and I could pack whatever I wanted. I don't really remember binge eating until I was old enough to drive at sixteen.

THERAPIST: So now what was going on when you were sixteen? Let's just kind of talk about that year, what was happening for you?

BARB: I was a sophomore in high school—this is so hard, it's so long ago. When I was sixteen and a half I met a guy that was twenty-three. And I was comfortable because his ex-wife was way fatter than me. I dated him pretty much until I was eighteen. I pretty much kept it a secret from my parents.

THERAPIST: But he was divorced?

BARB: Well, I think he was separated. He divorced while we were going out.

THERAPIST: What happened to the relationship?

BARB: He gave me a beautiful engagement ring, I remember, and I'm sure the engagement ring was because of my father's status because he was not really the type to give somebody a one-carat diamond ring. And we had been going out a long time and I got pregnant. And he'd come down and take me to lunch almost every day. There was no way I was going to tell my parents. And so I had an illegal abortion.

THERAPIST: How was it, thinking back about being pregnant, having the abortion, how did you manage your feelings about that during that time?

BARB: I don't even remember having feelings. I don't remember being sad about it, I just remember being relieved that I wasn't pregnant because my father would have died in this little town.

In this example, Barb's tendency to keep herself hidden in relationships and her difficulty in acknowledging feelings have emerged as prominent themes similar to the issues that were raised during the review of the current episode. The therapist begins to focus on her interpersonal style and its negative consequences that lead to binge eating.

BARB: Then I worked and worked. And then one day, I was twenty, somebody introduced me to this guy who was a co-worker. And I fell head over heels for this guy. I had not dated at all for almost two years. He was married, he had two children, he had a wife that was six months pregnant, and he was separated. And I fell head over heels for him and he fell head over heels for me. And he and I took off for Michigan. Moved as far away as we could and we lived together for four years. We told everybody we got married and we didn't. My parents to this day think I've been married twice. So then I was homesick, terribly, I just couldn't stand it.

THERAPIST: Now were you binge eating at that time when you were in Michigan?

BARB: I'm sure I was. I can remember eating on the bus.

THERAPIST: When in the process did you find yourself feeling homesick? Was that right away, or was it only after a period of time, or when you were aware of kind of having . . .

BARB: I think my "husband" was cheating on me then because he was working with another friend and he used to tell me about our friends, that her husband cheated on her terribly at work. And I think maybe it might have been him and I started to feel very insecure and I just wanted to get home. I can remember binge eating in Michigan because he wouldn't come home until late at night, he worked as a salesman. And I can remember food being my only friend, food and television, until he walked through the door and then I never ate.

THERAPIST: And then it was more in some respects to have the uncertainty or the loneliness or just kind of not knowing what's going on.

BARB: Not knowing what's going on, but I always believed what he told me because I wanted to.

THERAPIST: You needed to be connected. One thing that you talked about at least early on was a pattern of secretiveness. And tell me about that because it seems like even pretty early on you kind of got into this habit of . . .

BARB: My whole life I never ate in front of people, ever.

THERAPIST: Well, not just with your eating but just with other things as well, not telling your family about your first relationship, not telling them that you were pregnant, not telling them about Michigan. Even to the point where you were with your husband for twenty-two years and you worked to kind of keep it a secret. It seems that these times were also times when you were struggling more with your binge eating. Are you seeing that connection?

BARB: I never really thought about it until this second, never.

After a review of the past interpersonal functioning, the therapist switches to a review of current interpersonal functioning. The goal of this section of the interview is to continue helping patients make meaningful connections among their current functioning, significant interpersonal events, and the disorder itself. In addition, the therapist will be considering a number of ideas about potential goal areas to assist patients in making changes in their interpersonal problem areas.

REVIEWING CURRENT
INTERPERSONAL FUNCTIONING

THERAPIST: Now let's review your relationship with your husband.

BARB: I met my husband at the local town fair. I was twenty-seven. And he went away for about three weeks to get his kids, he had three children by a previous marriage. When he came back we were going to be married and I got pregnant. I can remember telling my mother after the marriage that I had just found out I was pregnant. That was all a lie because I knew I was pregnant when we got married.

THERAPIST: Didn't want to disappoint your parents?

BARB: Didn't want to disappoint them. . . .

THERAPIST: You talked earlier in the interview about hating him. . . .

BARB: Yeah, I hated him every, and I hated him every time he yelled at me. I hated the way he treated me. I hated him.

THERAPIST: And what did you do with all those feelings?

BARB: I put them into my son.

THERAPIST: You mean the hate? You mean . . . ?

BARB: No, the love.

THERAPIST: So what you did is that as he was being that way to you, you were just really trying to . . .

BARB: . . . the other way. And I did a heck of a job. I have a wonderful son.

THERAPIST: And what were you doing for yourself during that time?

BARB: (whispering) Nothing.

THERAPIST: And how was your eating during that time?

BARB: Bad. It was the heaviest I ever got. I was up to 265 pounds when I left the relationship.

THERAPIST: So while you were in the relationship with your husband, you just kept it all inside and you really channeled a lot of energy to your son. And then it sounds like you channeled a lot of that into a lot of activities and kept yourself . . .

BARB: I was the youth director of the church, a Den Mother. And that made it happy for me then.

THERAPIST: Yet you were doing a lot of things but then it sounds like, too, that was a time for you when you ended up with increased weight gain and binge eating.

BARB: Yes.

SUMMARIZING THE INTERPERSONAL INVENTORY

Toward the end of the interpersonal inventory, it is important for the therapist to summarize the interview in a manner that provides a transition between the fact-finding process and the collaborative establishment of treatment goals. Because the interpersonal inventory is conducted in this shortened format, it requires the therapist to move quickly into discussing the most important connections with the patient and, at times, to lead the patient into quite vulnerable domains. It is not uncommon for patients to feel emotionally overwhelmed, especially when the pregroup assessment and the interpersonal inventory are conducted within a day or two of each other. Therefore, it is important to take time within the context of the interpersonal inventory to provide a framework to help the patient understand how difficulties managing interpersonal relationships are related to an increase in symptoms. In the next portion of the interview, note that the patient seems to be making some connections but has not yet understood their relevance to her symptoms.

THERAPIST: I'm struck by the degree to which you tried to manage and keep everybody else feeling like everything's OK while holding on to all those feelings without telling anyone about your troubles. You really poured a lot into caring for your son, and maintaining this relationship where there was really no connection or intimacy. That takes a lot of effort.

BARB: A lot of energy. But I did it.

THERAPIST: You did. And so in many respects you can look back on that and say that you did that, but then I wonder, too, if during that time in terms of thinking about . . .

BARB: Sure, because I was proud of the fact that I could do it. I felt very successful in everything except my weight. And I had always succeeded at everything I ever, in every job I ran and with the . . .

THERAPIST: No, it's clear. And you've done extremely well.

BARB: Yes. And now I own my own business, and I'm very successful. And now I'm building a bigger one because we're going to move. I mean I'm very successful at whatever I do.

THERAPIST: This would probably be a good time to move into the next phase of what we need to talk about. I'm aware that the way in which you manage your feelings about your relationship, or lack of relationship, with others—that there may be some areas in which we might be able to help you out. Because it seems to me that oftentimes, granted, it's like you're doing so well but at what cost?

BARB: I would never say any of this to anybody, but I've never, not even my minister, you are the only person that knows.

THERAPIST: What do you mean, that knows what?

BARB: That I even cried when I talked about something.

THERAPIST: Do you just not let people know these things?

BARB: I guess.

THERAPIST: How has this been for you, talking here?

BARB: Fine, fine.

THERAPIST: And so have you felt . . .

BARB: As long as you don't think I'm weird for crying.

THERAPIST: Heavens, no. It does feel like you've really tapped into a lot of feelings since we've talked about a number of things. I think that part of it, too, might be that most of your life you've really done a pretty good job keeping people from knowing very much about what you're thinking or feeling. And that has to affect the quality of your connection to others.

BARB: Right. And I know you're going to find it out, and it's very hard for me.

THERAPIST: But I think that's going to be worthwhile, and I appreciate your willingness to explore that. Because again, in many respects, although you've done a good job not disappointing people, in many respects it sounds like you've used food, binge eating over the years, as a way to hold things together. Because you can't continue to live, and I'm not using the word *deception* in a negative way, but it's like the degrees to which you've had to deceive in order to be able to manage . . .

BARB: Hundreds of people I've deceived.

THERAPIST: It's a heavy burden because you consider yourself a good person and you do the right thing and you're honest. But yet the level at which you have to keep things held together, my hunch is that's where the food issue comes in. You don't like conflicts and you have difficulty being yourself with others, letting others know you, so you try to skirt that or try to make peace and not let anybody be disappointed in you. And it seems like that's where food comes in. It calms you down, relaxes you, stuffs things away, you know, so you don't have to think about anything. Maybe that's why it's hard for you to have any downtime because as soon as you do, it's almost as if too many things get to you . . . so if you keep busy all the time you're okay.

BARB: Yeah, it could be.

ESTABLISHING TARGET GOALS

Target goals are developed by the clinician in collaboration with the patient. It is important for the therapist to frame these goals within the context of the data gathered during the interview rather than on the basis of general clinical impressions. It is more likely, in any case, that patients will collaboratively accept goals based on the interview data. Another way the therapist can support goals is by reviewing with patients the specific responses on questionnaires that they themselves have completed. In addition, target goals can be rated for severity by the patient before treatment begins.

In later sessions, these goals can be rated in terms of relevance to what has been worked on in therapy, and improvement. Goals that are altered as treatment progresses may reflect a record of deepening self-understanding. The interpersonal patterns and subsequent goals that are revealed within the context of the interview will specifically be used during the first phase of IPT-G.

One way to begin the process of establishing goals is to ask patients whether they have made any connections during the interview and thought of any goals that they would like to work on. Alternatively, the therapist can share some of his or her own thoughts about the interview, suggest some goals to the patient, and assess with the patient whether they seem accurate based on the information shared. At this point in the interview, the therapist can also explain that the goals will be written down on paper, and that the patient will be asked for feedback on them during the first few sessions of the group. In our continuing example below, the therapist uses the interview data to begin formulating treatment goals:

THERAPIST: One of goals that I've been thinking about, as we've been talking, is that it really would be important for you to start letting people know more about some of the things that are going on, what you're thinking and feeling. You hold on to those too much. The pattern that you've established throughout the years is that if something's going on, you don't want to disappoint anybody or cause any conflict, and so you don't say anything or skirt it or spin a story about it. But yet you end up holding onto it, and it has an effect. People don't get to know you, and you lose connections to others. And you've been doing it for years. Specifically, it seems that the times when you keep things to yourself, even now with your boyfriend, is when you find yourself binge eating.

BARB: You're right, I have done that for years.

THERAPIST: Also, because of your tendency to hide things and maintain an appearance that everything is OK, people seek you out because you appear really calm, happy-go-lucky, and stable. But the more you work to keep things stable, the more you become an anchor for other people. Then there's nobody that's holding you together but you and food.

BARB: Right.

THERAPIST: Another part of the picture is that it sounds like you often shut off what you're experiencing even from yourself. You're trying to keep so many things together that you're not being mindful of what's happening with you because you're worried about what's happening with everybody else. So taking time to experience yourself and the issues going on, especially in your relationships, will be important. If you can learn to do that, you're less likely to be using food to do it. Now, as we've been talking, is there anything else that's come up that you think would be worthwhile to work on or that you find that's more associated or connected with your eating? Other than what we've kind of talked about?

BARB: Like what we've talked about, I never really realized that's what it was. It makes a lot of sense to me.

THERAPIST: Do you think it would be worthwhile pursuing these sorts of goals?

BARB: Uh-huh.

THERAPIST: All right. So the group will be able to help you do that, and I think it will be possible.

As the therapist collaboratively identifies goals with the patient, it is critical that these goals be meaningfully linked to the problem area (e.g., interpersonal deficits in Barb's case) as well as specific and attainable given the patients' inter- and intrapersonal dynamics and social networks. Another helpful strategy, when writing down the patients' goals (which we strongly encourage), is to use the same language and phrasing that were used during the session. In addition, it is helpful to anchor the goals in the context of interpersonal examples. In doing so, the therapist ensures that the goals of all patients become personal and relevant to their work over the course of the group. These goals should be expressed in such a way that they focus on the important changes that patients can begin to make in their outside social networks. They should also link the patients' work in the group with these changes. (See following example.)

EXAMPLES OF A PATIENT'S GOALS RELATED TO BINGE EATING FOR THE IPT PROBLEM AREA OR INTERPERSONAL DEFICITS

1. During the interview you shared that over the years you have kept many secrets and, in the process, have kept your thoughts and feelings hidden inside. You mentioned that you have done this to protect people you care about (for example, your father and your son) and to protect yourself from having conflict with others. Your difficulty in communicating effectively and directly has made it difficult for you to manage conflict. From the time since this began, binge eating has been one way for you to manage the pressure of keeping yourself hidden or distant in relationships.

Goal: In order for you to recover from your binge eating, it will be very important for you to begin to share your thoughts and feelings (both good and bad) with the important people in your life, such as your son and your boyfriend. This will ultimately bring you closer, though the others will have to get used to dealing with a "new you." Use the group as a place to practice talking about your life and the issues you are trying to deal with. As you become more comfortable doing this, you will be less likely to use food as a way to keep your feelings inside.

2. You also mentioned that you have spent a good part of your life caring for and taking care of others (your son, your relationships, your organizations, your customers). Your overall competence has led people to come to you for support or to take on extra tasks that add to your already busy schedule.

Goal: In order to recover from your binge eating it will be important for you to develop techniques for saying "no." This means that you will need to challenge the guilt you experience if you don't immediately accept more responsibilities and your fears that others will not like you if you refuse. This cycle of self-denial and excessive responsibility appears to have had a negative effect on your relationships. Addressing this pattern will free up time for yourself, and doing nice things for yourself would be a good way to start. As you give yourself priority, you will be less likely to need to use food to nurture yourself. The group will provide a good opportunity to discuss ways of addressing this goal and then to keep the group informed as to how it is progressing.

3. During our meeting you talked about having a difficult time identifying your thoughts and feelings, especially times when you binge eat. We know that many individuals who struggle with binge eating also have problems identifying just what is going on inside. This makes it hard to address the important interpersonal issues. Food can be calming and soothing. The more aware you can be about your thoughts and feelings, the less likely you will need to use food as a way to manage them. Over the years, your binge eating has been one way that you have tried to take care of yourself. Unfortunately, this strategy has not been very successful and has led to just the opposite—your continuing to feel out of control and demoralized. By identifying what is triggering the desire to eat, you will become better able to address those issues directly.

Goal: When you begin to binge eat or feel out of control with your eating, stop and check in with yourself by asking "What's going on?

What's the interpersonal issue that triggered this? How has it made me feel? What can I do to address the situation?" This may be difficult at first, so both inside and outside of the group try to be mindful of upset states and address the underlying issues and feelings as they come up—in the moment. As you become better able to do this, you will be less likely to use food to blanket your distress.

CASE EXAMPLES INVOLVING TYPICAL PATIENT GOALS RELATED TO THE IPT PROBLEM AREAS FOR DEPRESSION

PROBLEM AREA: GRIEF

The death of your wife four years ago was a very difficult time. Her lengthy illness with cancer occupied a great deal of your time and energy, and this was complicated by her demanding nature. From your description it appears that the event of her actual death was not really addressed. You looked after all the funeral arrangements and then returned directly to work. You have acted responsibly in caring for your three young children since then, though perhaps this focus also provided a diversion from dealing with both the grief and the anger you describe experiencing.

Goal: An unresolved grief reaction is a common trigger for depression. You will need to revisit the time around your wife's death and let yourself go back in time to reexperience all that was happening. This will be a complicated but important task. On the one hand you adored your wife, but on the other her rather forceful personality became increasingly demanding during her illness. This process of working through the grief may be helped by going through any pictures or letters you might have from your wife and also talking to good friends who were involved at the time. You might also think of reconnecting with her by visiting her grave, a task that you have been avoiding. The group will provide an opportunity to talk about your wife from both the positive and not-so-positive perspectives and give you an opportunity to let yourself grieve.

PROBLEM AREA:
INTERPERSONAL DISPUTES

You describe your current depression as being directly connected to a lengthy intimate relationship about which you feel quite ambivalent. On the one hand, you question whether your partner will allow it to progress from its present state into a full and committed relationship; on the other, you find yourself quite dependent on the relationship to fulfill your legitimate emotional needs for a close bond with someone. You feel that this impasse affects your feelings about yourself and your future.

Goal: No one can make this decision for you, but it is important that the situation be brought to a head—by either achieving a commitment for a future with your partner or resolving that the relationship must end. It is important to get off the stuck position in which you have felt yourself trapped for several years. The group will provide an opportunity to explore the basis of this relationship and especially the emotions it creates within you. Talking about the implications of the two alternatives and getting ideas from others in the group may help you in your decision.

PROBLEM AREA: ROLE TRANSITION

You see yourself as somewhat sheltered and naive and feel very much under parental supervision even though your parents live abroad. You are acutely aware that your parents' admonitions are always in your mind, and you describe these negative messages as continually reinforcing your depression. While you do not wish to discontinue connections with your parents, you feel the current ways of interacting are damaging to you. You want to move on to make your own decisions in your life.

Goal: Your goal is to begin setting up some clear boundaries with your parents. This will entail standing up for yourself and setting limits on the influence of your parents, so that you are not as enmeshed in their expectations (or at least your ideas of their expectations). Part of this task is to come to terms with just how emotional you feel about this situation, but your feelings are kept under tight control. The group will provide an opportunity to talk about these issues, including your emotions as you experience them in the group, and to develop strategies that allow you to become less reactive to your parents and increase your social network to include more peer relationships.

PROBLEM AREA: INTERPERSONAL DEFICITS

You describe yourself as quite socially isolated even though you have many potential creative interests. From your descriptions, you can be quite open and friendly in the workplace, but this changes immediately when you leave work. Depression generally responds to an increase in interpersonal social contact.

Goal: It would be helpful to become more actively involved in social organizations associated with your interests. Your membership would be an opportunity to talk to others and perhaps develop some ongoing friendships. It would also be an opportunity to decrease your anxiety about how people might see you and whether that corresponds to your view that you are ugly. It will be important to discuss this goal with the group and use the group sessions themselves to monitor efforts to become more involved and self-disclosing.

PREPARING FOR GROUP WORK

The final task in the pregroup interview involves preparing patients for the group treatment. As demonstrated in earlier examples, throughout the interview regular connections will be made between the historical material being elicited and how it might be addressed in the group. It is helpful to encourage patients to think of the group as an "interpersonal laboratory" where ties to others can develop, where naturally occurring "impasses" in the formation of relationships can be examined in detail, and where patients can experiment with new approaches to handling interpersonal problems. Finally, it is helpful to describe the social skills that patients learn while participating in a group and to stress that a main goal of the group is to help them apply these skills to their outside social lives. These include such interpersonal skills as giving or receiving support from others, clarification of interpersonal issues, interpersonal confrontation, honest communication, and expression of feelings.

When conducting the interpersonal inventory, the therapist can use the interview to demonstrate how the group will work by treating this individual session like a "mini-group." Specifically, as the patient's disturbed patterns of relating in his or her current social network are identified, the therapist can begin to anticipate with the patient how these patterns are likely to emerge in the context of the therapy group. For patients with interpersonal deficits, for example, the therapist may explain how, when they describe distressing experiences, they use language that is somewhat vague and intellectualized—a verbal style that may confuse listeners and contribute to feeling misunderstood. Following this "in-session observation," the therapist can elicit the patient's reactions to such feedback and explore what it will be like to receive similar feedback in the group. This technique can be quite useful for helping patients understand how the group will work and how elements of their interpersonal style may contribute to their difficulties in relationships.

A simple introduction to how therapy groups work is helpful, especially when provided in the form of a handout, as it gives each patient an opportunity to ask questions about the nature of the group experience. (A model handout can be found in Appendix C.) This handout should be given to the patient at the first pregroup meeting so that it can be read at leisure and away from the pressure of a face-to-face interview. A few minutes at the last pregroup meeting should be devoted to reviewing it and answering any questions or addressing any apprehensions that the patient might have. And the material in the handout should be quietly reinforced in early sessions of the group itself. It is useful to emphasize that there is sound clinical evidence indicating that psychotherapy in a group setting is as effective as individual psychotherapy. The basic group rules should also be reviewed, particularly the one regarding confidentiality.

Checklist for Pregroup Interviews

1. Discuss chief complaint and symptoms/syndrome.
2. Obtain history of symptoms.
3. Assign patient the "sick role."
4. Establish whether or not there is a history of prior treatments for the disorder or other psychiatric problems.
5. Assess patient's expectations about psychotherapy.
6. Reassure patient about positive prognosis.
7. Explain IPT and its basic assumptions.
8. Complete an interpersonal inventory (i.e., a detailed review of important relationships):
   - Review past interpersonal functioning (e.g., family, school, social life).
   - Examine *current* interpersonal functioning (e.g., family, work, social life).
   - Identify the interpersonal precipitants of episodes of symptoms.
9. Translate symptoms into an interpersonal context.
10. Explain IPT techniques.
11. Contract for administrative details (i.e., length of sessions, frequency, duration of treatment, appointment times).
12. Provide feedback to patient regarding general understanding of IPT problem area(s), interpersonal target goals, and interpersonal triggers.
13. Collaborate on a contract regarding the treatment goals.
14. Explain tasks in working toward treatment goals.

Checklist of Issues to Be
Addressed Concerning the Group

1. Discuss group structure (i.e., size of group, duration of meetings, time boundaries).
2. Discuss attendance and punctuality.
3. Discuss confidentiality.
4. Discuss presence of a process observer, if indicated.
5. Explain patient/therapist roles.
6. Using various examples, describe the group as an "interpersonal laboratory"—that is, as a place to
   - work on relationship difficulties.
   - learn from other group members.
   - recognize and accept the opinions, feelings, and needs of other members.
   - discover that general learning will come from becoming actively involved in the group.
7. Discuss the importance of transferring newly learned skills to outside social life.
8. Explain that the influence of early childhood experience is recognized as significant, but that the treatment is focused on the present and applied to the patients' current social lives.
9. Forewarn patients about the shift from individual therapist to group, and explain that they will learn from the group and have less direct interaction with the therapist.
10. Discuss the possibility that some participants may want to drop out within the first few sessions, and explain that it is important to talk about such feelings with the group because others may be feeling the same way.

SUMMARY

There are many tasks to be completed during the individual pre-group meetings. Developing an adequate database for diagnosis and suitability for the intended group is a first priority. Identifying the primary problem area and collaboratively establishing treatment goals are also extremely important for both the therapist and the patient during this first phase of IPT-G. Even more important are the connections that the therapist and patient make about the patient's interpersonal problems and the onset or maintenance of his or her disorder. These critical connections form the foundation of the patient's goals and provide a road map for making the necessary changes that will lead to a recovery. Forging these connections during the pregroup interviews also helps establish a strong working alliance and quickly establishes the credibility of the treatment and the expertise of the therapist. Indeed, our collective experience suggests that the better patients are able to grasp the interpersonal connections to the onset and/or maintenance of their disorder, the better they are able to make use of the first phase of IPT-G.

NOTES

1. In the NIMH study for BED (Wilfley et al., 1999), the pregroup interview was conducted during a two-hour session. The paper-and-pencil assessments and structured clinical assessments were conducted over several days prior to the pregroup meeting.

PART THREE
THE GROUP

CHAPTER 4

The Initial Phase

The task of the initial phase of treatment is to refine and consolidate at a group level the tasks introduced in the individual pregroup interviews. Each step of the transition from the individual meetings to the group process will build on the prior step. The group members are primed during the individual interviews to begin work on their interpersonal problem areas. By helping members to make preliminary connections between their symptoms and relationship difficulties, the therapist sets in motion a degree of productive momentum. The therapist then amplifies and continues this momentum as members begin to learn to work together as a group. Sessions 1 to 5 comprise IPT-G's initial phase, during which the therapist has the following overall objectives:

- to cultivate positive group norms and group cohesion;
- to emphasize the commonality of symptoms and how they will be addressed;
- to educate the members about IPT-G theory and their role in treatment;
- to review the interpersonal inventory of each group member and link his or her symptoms to the interpersonal context; and
- to consolidate the principal problem area and establish a treatment contract.

Whereas longer-term groups encourage members to generate their own working norms over time, IPT's short-term model mandates that the therapist take the initiative in establishing positive group norms straightaway. The over-arching aim is to ensure that the group begins its formation around a focus on the problematic issues; in this way, members are encouraged to commit to work with each other on individual target goals right away. It is essential that the therapist be actively involved in these initial sessions to ensure that the group is anchored in the IPT framework. Another key task is to ensure that the group functions as a group—not as people receiving individual therapy in a group format. As the treatment progresses, and the members learn the rules of the group, they can become more responsible for choosing relevant material to discuss, while the therapist can become less directive.

In sessions 1 and 2, the therapist is charged with simultaneously cultivating positive group cohesion—the glue that transforms various individuals into a functional group (see Chapter 2)—and orienting the group toward IPT treatment principles and processes. In sessions 3 to 5, members delineate specific target goals and begin to take steps toward change.

SESSION 1: GETTING STARTED

LAYING THE GROUNDWORK

As with all groups, the members' first connection is with the therapist. Indeed, in session 1, members will frequently direct all communication to the therapist with whom they have developed some degree of trust. The most effective way to advance a group sense of acceptance and trust is through the promotion of member-to-member interaction. Therefore, a basic task of this session is to introduce the members to each other and to begin to build norms that facilitate working as a group on the problem areas discussed in the individual pregroup interviews.

Once all the members have shared names, the group therapist needs to reiterate the specific diagnosis that has brought the group together. As noted in earlier chapters, an important component here is giving members what is technically known in the social psychology literature as the "sick role" while also instilling hope and confidence about treatment. The symptom review, diagnosis, and description of the type and course of treatment all function to give the group member this role. It is important to describe the recovery process, because it sets up the expectation that the sick role is undesirable and should be relinquished as soon as possible. Implicitly the message is that the member has a responsibility in getting better. Although this information has been conveyed to some extent in the pregroup interviews, saying it again to the group will have the effect of helping everyone to join around the expectation of working together and getting better.

It is also helpful to provide members with a statement about the general direction of the group structure throughout the upcoming weeks. By doing so, the therapist will demystify the therapeutic process and facilitate the building of positive norms and cohesion, both part of a well-functioning group. Following are excerpts from a first session that illustrate how a therapist might introduce these initial fundamental components. For the purpose of general utilization, the diagnosis is not specified. In an actual group, however, the therapist would adapt these comments to a specific diagnosis such as depression or binge eating.

INTRODUCTIONS

THERAPIST: Welcome everyone. I know we're all looking forward to getting going; you've all been through the same sequence of questionnaires and interviews. Let's start off with introductions and have each of you introduce yourself. We'll come back later in the group to hear more about everyone after we cover some preliminary tasks.

REITERATING THE DIAGNOSIS
AND EXPLAINING IPT TREATMENT

THERAPIST: As we mentioned before to each of you, everyone in
the group has a diagnosis of binge eating, a common disorder
affecting 30 percent of overweight individuals seeking treatment. This group is one treatment that has been found to be effective in helping people to recover. Research has shown that
the progress people make here continues even after the group
ends. Most members see changes in their eating symptoms and
notice better interpersonal relations by the end of treatment.

The purpose of the interpersonal group is for each of you to
work hard to focus in on relationships and on feelings that
have typically been associated with your binge eating. We have
identified times with you when you're most likely to struggle
with difficult symptoms. In formulating your goals, we tried to
draw some of the same connections that each of you had identified when we met in the initial interview. The intent over the
next few months is to be working actively on those goals and to
make changes. I encouraged a lot of you in the pregroup meeting to go ahead and start doing some thinking, some reflecting,
and to stop and process your feelings.

EDUCATING ABOUT GROUP STRUCTURE

THERAPIST: We will be meeting for twenty weeks for an hour and
a half each time. The first few minutes and the last ten to fifteen
minutes of each group will be reserved for check-in/wrap-up.
We can break the treatment down probably into three kinds of
discrete periods. This session we're going to be spending time
getting to know one another. But, also, these first five sessions
are a real opportunity for you to "try on" the goals that we've
initially formulated based on our contact with you. We expect
that over the next five weeks you may have changes that you
want to make, or areas where we didn't quite exactly meet the

goal that you were thinking about. If it's not working, we want
to know about it.

Sessions 6 to 16 comprise the work stage, the time when we're
going to be actively working and people will begin to make
many changes. You're going to notice changes in your symptoms, in your outside life, in how you're relating with other
people, and in how you're relating with each other. And that is
all a part of the process.

The final transition sessions, from 17 to 20, make up the last
phase, when we'll be wrapping things up and helping people
to solidify what they've learned and to get prepared for the end
of the group. We have a lot of time and we will be able to do a
lot of work in that twenty-week period.

Collaborating on Goals

Formulation of goals occurs in a collaborative manner in the pregroup interviews or intake meetings. By the first group session, members need to receive a clear written summary of their goals (or
preliminary treatment plan) based on these interviews. In the following excerpt of session 1, members are encouraged to take their target
goals—developed in terms of problem area, specific interpersonal
events, or problematic relationships—and rethink them to see if they
"fit." Note that the members and the therapist work together on this
significant aspect of treatment:

THERAPIST: As for your goals that we passed back to you, hold
onto them. If you feel like you've written what you wanted to
write, and you've given your feedback, we'll take them. If not,
from tonight's session, go through those with a fine-toothed
comb. Really think about having them fit for you. We'll be getting your comments on those over the next several weeks.
Then we'll reconfigure them and give them back to you by session 6. That will be our working document for the remainder of
treatment.

It is imperative for there to be agreement between the therapist and the group members about goals. If such agreement is lacking, a group member may show his or her dissatisfaction by missing sessions, not participating in the group, or dropping out.

GROUP COHESION

Building mutual cooperation and support among members is central to the group's development. As members begin to discuss their reasons for joining the group and reveal their initial target goals, the therapists must at the same time endeavor to shape a cohesive group. Group therapists can foster cohesion by reinforcing three supportive therapeutic factors that emerge in the early stages of all groups: universality, acceptance, and altruism. Much of this work can be done by underlining interactions in these three areas when they occur. In this excerpt from session 1, the therapist emphasizes similarities among group members:

> CO-THERAPIST: I was thinking now is a good time to get reactions and comments from people. I noticed some themes that people seemed in agreement about. I was struck by the similarity in what each of you are bringing here. And I think that in many ways you'll be able to use that, and not feel so isolated at least.
> CAROLINE: Yeah, it is nice to know I'm not the only one that feels this way. I don't have children and yet some of the things that I hear people saying about their feelings and their relationships with their children are very similar to feelings that I've had with my husband, with other people in my life. So I guess the emotions are the same. In some cases I identify with everyone and I think about ways that I've felt the same.

Another way to underscore similarities is to ask group members how they are affected by another member's discussion. In this way, common issues take shape and members are encouraged to join forces in working on goals:

THERAPIST: As Jeanne talks, are others connecting in with what she is saying? You're nodding your head. . . .

Therapists need to encourage all members to be involved in every session, especially silent members, who may need to be brought in early with gentle encouragement. Altruistic events can be commented on as examples of helpful interactions. As they begin to establish group unity, members will become more likely to trust each other and the group process itself. This type of environment will also make it easier for members to take tentative steps toward self-disclosure.

DISCUSSING THE PROBLEM AREAS

In the first session, the therapist quite actively encourages and guides members to elaborate on their previously formulated problem areas and associated target goals. Such elaboration is a priority when building the foundation of the IPT framework. If a group member is struggling, the therapist can gently remind him or her of issues discussed and connections made during pregroup interviews that seem relevant to the current discussion. The therapist can also use pregroup information to join members by highlighting mutual issues, thus adding to feelings of universality.

During this phase of the group, the therapist also needs to help members gain a fuller understanding of the ways in which their symptoms are linked to their difficulties in managing relationships. Given an adequate assessment, most members will arrive at the first session with a nascent awareness of this connection. Nearly all will need continued guidance to gain a working understanding of this relationship, to refine target goals, and to develop strategies for change.

Another challenge for the therapist is to build what is in fact personal work into a structure that can facilitate group interaction. The objective is to avoid establishing a format whereby the therapist attends to individuals in turn with decreasing responsibility for group interaction. A helpful strategy here is to consistently encourage members to share comments or to reveal their own connections to another group member's story.

The following is an excerpt taken from a first group of IPT-G for depression in which the therapist begins by orienting the members to the process of sharing a little about themselves and their goals. Notice how the therapist assists Samantha by bringing in information from the pregroup interviews, guides her to clarify her goals in the area of interpersonal deficits, and encourages others to join the discussion:

THERAPIST: Today you will begin to communicate with people you don't know and find out what it's like to be in a group. Talk a little bit about who you are and what brings you here. And then, if you feel like you can, maybe share a little bit about some of the goals that you have set for yourself or some of the things that you think you are going to be interested in working on over the next twenty weeks.

Next session, we will start talking more about the important people in your life and the people that you're really needing to make changes with. So, that's how we'll have things unfold over at least the next couple of sessions. Again, as things come up, and as issues come up with the goals, we'll want to talk about that with you. Who would like to start?

SAMANTHA: I will. My name's Samantha. I've been a secretary for many years. I have a great husband, a terrific little toddler. So, externally, everything just seems great, but I've been really depressed. I just got the group goals as I was leaving for tonight's session. I didn't really get to look at them except for at the traffic lights.

THERAPIST: I think one of the things that we had talked about being important [in the pregroup interviews] was what other group members have been talking about today, about not feeling validated. And I think that was one of the things that you had talked about, too. So not being validated by your parents and then not feeling like you've been able to let other people give you positive feedback or say good things about you, especially even your husband. . . .

SAMANTHA: Yeah.

THERAPIST: That seemed like a real important connection.

SAMANTHA: It was. Just after I had met with you, it was just—I sat out in my car and I cried. I've thought about it a lot since I met with you both. It touched on things. And I mean I've had therapy for years, and nothing ever struck a chord for me like it did in my session with you both.

THERAPIST: Also, I think you mentioned difficulties in your work situation as well. You find yourself feeling frustrated, not feeling like you have the right to speak up.

SAMANTHA: Right.

THERAPIST: Right. And I think—Caroline, you had mentioned that, too, not feeling like you had the right to express yourself.

CAROLINE: For me it is more with my family, not so much work situations. I don't want to hurt anyone's feelings so I tend to keep it to myself. I don't want to feel like a burden.

THERAPIST: . . . so, feeling it is not OK to share your feelings.

SAMANTHA: . . . uh, that's creating a problem more and more within myself and in my relationships.

CAROLINE: For me too. It is so hard, though, to do that.

THERAPIST: Is anyone else connecting with this issue?

In a first meeting involving members with binge eating disorder, Tammy introduces herself and is encouraged to discuss her goals and difficulties managing her relationships. As with Samantha, Tammy's primary problem area is interpersonal deficits. Observe that the therapist handles the patient's initial complaint—that she doesn't know how to approach her goals—by helping her to clarify how her symptoms of binge eating are related to the way that she manages her intimate relationships. The therapist also prompts her to consider the issues she raised in the pregroup interviews. Other members are urged to participate in this exploration as well:

TAMMY: Okay. I'm Tammy; I'm divorced. I have two dogs, no kids. I retired after thirty years as a market analyst and now have my own businesses. I've been eating to compensate for something that's been wrong with me since I was in high school and reading self-help books to find out what was wrong with me. My father was very verbally and physically abusive. So, after watching the model that my mother set, silence was the safest way to approach things, and ultimately eating was the way to put the lid on it. The first goal on my sheet, I mean I can't remember off the top of my head what it was, but it's that I had no clue how I was going to approach that. That's why I feel I need to seek help to get feedback.

THERAPIST: Is your dad still alive?

TAMMY: Yes, my parents are still alive. The relationship is improved with my dad. He almost died a couple of years ago. When he came out of the hospital, he was just so grateful to be back. The tenderness that I saw, I'd never seen before. Now he doesn't let us go without saying I love you. And it's like, yeah, this is what I want. You know, it's not what the little kid in me needed so much, but it's certainly what I as an adult need from my dad and it's helped me to accept that love. Because it was like, I was going to be angry and never forgive you and now, sort of, I can let some of that in.

THERAPIST: So, it is nice that the relationship has really taken a turn. I think that's been important. I think one of the things you shared with us, though, is the style of pushing your feelings away, keeping some of that tucked away.

TAMMY: Right.

THERAPIST: And that your relationships end up getting derailed at times in that way. And that's been problematic and troublesome for you.

TAMMY: Right, because when I enter a relationship, it's "Who does that person want me to be?" and "If I can be that person, they'll love me." And I'm very conflict avoiding so I just try to shut down, back off, you know, keep the water calm.

THERAPIST: Well, I think that's one of the goals for you: to really spend some time and think and talk about that. What are other people's thoughts about what Tammy has been saying?

TODD: I was thinking as she was talking that I do that too . . . especially when I am dating. So, I've stopped dating. But I'm getting more isolated. And that's a problem.

This session continued as group members talked further about their target goals.

WRAP-UP

The therapist asks for comments at the end of each session during what is known as the wrap-up. This process is helpful as a way of gauging each member's involvement and emotional state. Sometimes, members become quite aroused emotionally during the session; in such cases they can use this brief check-in as a way to gather themselves before leaving. In the following example, notice how the therapist acknowledges the group member's concern without encouraging further disclosure at this time:

THERAPIST: We've got just a few minutes left and I wanted to wrap things up and check in with people about how things went and how you feel, even tonight. Any thoughts or feelings, Sam, about how the first group went for you?

SAM: I think it went very well. There are still some issues that I'm hiding . . . that I am sure will come out.

THERAPIST: I'm sure that's true.

SAM: . . . that I haven't talked to even my medical doctor about and a lot of my family. Not that I'm physically sick, but some things that I have done that he probably needs to know about in my past that I'm still hiding that I'll talk about when I feel comfortable.

THERAPIST: Well, I think that part of the process, too, is getting to a place where you feel more comfortable. How has it gone today for others?

It is clear that Sam will need time in the next session to begin to share the concerns he has mentioned during the last fifteen minutes of this session. The therapist needs to be sure that this follow-up does indeed take place.

SUMMARY

There are many points to raise in this first session. The therapist will need to be diligent in covering each. The ideas introduced here can be reviewed in session 2 as needed. You have done your job as therapist if you are successful in eliciting a response from all of the members about their initial goals and if the members begin to learn a little about each other and the commonality of their symptoms. The main objective in this first group is to help members join the group without overdisclosing. Given the extensive pregroup preparation and goal formulation in IPT-G, it is not uncommon for members to come "charging out of the gate" during the first session. When this phenomenon occurs, the therapist can educate the group about it and encourage members to go slowly at first as there will be plenty of time for them to get to know one another. When the therapist allows a member to overdisclose in the first session, other members will assume that this is how they are supposed to share as well, and they may become uncomfortable and anxious. (See Table 4.1 for a summary checklist covering session 1.)

SESSION 2: THE ROLE OF MEMBERS

At the start of session 2, the therapists can suggest that members reintroduce themselves and raise any questions they may have

TABLE 4.1   Summary Checklist for Session 1

Therapist Tasks

1. Start and end group on time.
2. Welcome and introduce members.
3. Cultivate positive group norms and cohesion:
   - Reiterate the common diagnosis, and generate the expectatin of recovery.
   - Educate about IPT treatment, group structure, and process issues.
   - Encourage all members to join in the discussion of interpersonal problem areas and associated target goals, using information gleaned in pregroup interviews.
   - Begin to facilitate member self-disclosure.

Individual Patient Tasks

1. Introduce self (including details regarding reason for joining group, work stress, activities, and significant others).
2. Begin to understand IPT treatment structure and group process.
3. Develop feelings of connection to other members.
4. Reveal and begin to clarify initial target goals.
5. Perceive an expectation of recovery.

about the first group. From this discussion, the group therapists will be able to evaluate the extent to which members need to be reoriented to the group work. It is particularly valuable at this stage to teach members their role in IPT-G—to explain that they should let the therapist know if they are struggling, are not "getting it," or feel minor irritations about the group or its members. Group members are to play an active role in deciding where to go in the sessions, as long as they are maintaining a current focus on treatment goals. These guidelines can be mentioned by the therapist as an introductory comment at the start of session 2 and inserted thereafter as needed:

THERAPIST: We want to mention a few things about your role as a member. There may be times you feel uncomfortable in the group sessions and aren't sure why, or feel yourself withdrawing because of the topic being discussed. It will be important for you to bring this up rather than "shut down." We'll be active and give some structure, but it is also up to you to decide where things will go in the sessions and initiate these. We don't spend as much time focusing in on symptoms, though we are interested in how your involvement in the group and working toward your goals is affecting them.

Feeling States

A requisite therapist task introduced in session 2 is to emphasize the value of noticing feeling states both inside and outside of group. It is advantageous to teach members this skill early on as it encourages an awareness of internal reactions and promotes an understanding of how these reactions can affect their interpersonal relationships and impact symptoms. In the following excerpt from session 2 of a group for members with binge eating disorder, Mark begins to make a connection between his feelings and his symptoms. The therapist then encourages all group members to recognize and acknowledge their feelings and to begin to understand them in terms of the interpersonal context:

> MARK: What I've realized is that I get a negative feeling. It could be over a lot of things. But it gets to a point where I shift into overdrive, and my car will drive right into Jack in the Box. And I know that I'm shut down. I have to deal with it on a different level other than eating it. Because that's what I do, I eat it, to numb myself as you said. And whatever makes me get that way, whether it's my lack of sex life or whatever, I have to look at that.
>
> THERAPIST: That is one of the things we wanted to get you all started on: being thoughtful about what you are doing during the day and when you are binge eating. Be aware of when you find yourself "shifting." Did you just have an uncomfortable interaction with a co-worker? Were you thinking about some difficulty in a relationship? You may have found yourself shutting off in here tonight or cutting off in a way to be able to manage the relationships in here. Or, as things unfold, you may find that happening. And when it does, this is a marvelous time to bring it up, do something about it.

The group therapists need to recognize when members are withdrawing from the group interaction. Most likely, the members are reacting to something in the group that has triggered an internal response that they may have difficulty identifying and/or expressing. In the following example taken from a group with members diagnosed with major depression, the therapist is aware of a change in a group member. As the therapist facilitates acknowledgment of internal feelings, the member is able to address a troublesome interpersonal exchange:

> A group member fell silent during an early session. The therapist became aware of this and thought back quickly to when it developed. The withdrawal seemed to have occurred after a mild interaction with another member when the silent member was told that she resembled the other member's mother. Earlier, this mother had been described in negative terms. The therapist noted the member's silence and asked gently what she was experiencing. With great hesitation the member revealed that she had begun to wonder if she should be in the group because it would upset the other member. She began to cry and stated her perception that she could never really be accepted because of her inadequacies. The group quickly responded to reengage her and pointed out that she had every right to find out what the comment implied. This served as the initial trigger to begin to address the way she manages relationships by becoming nonassertive and compliant.

INTERPERSONAL REVIEW

Following the review of target goals in session 1, the therapist uses session 2 to guide the group's efforts toward revealing more about their significant relationships or lack thereof. The interpersonal review contributes to the IPT framework in a number of ways and often follows easily from the discussion of goals, as the two are linked. As members discuss these relationships, they become more attuned to their expectations about others and the associated feelings. This insight places them in a better position to determine the changes they would like to see. Additionally, it sets each group member in an interpersonal context, creating a greater depth of understanding among members. Increased cohesion may result as members recognize similar struggles in relationships. This fuller picture will also help members to support each other in modifying and applying goals.

By session 2, the pregroup preparation and initial review of target goals in session 1 will have led to discussion among some members about the ways in which they have begun to apply new approaches to their problem areas. By highlighting these efforts, the therapist can assist other members in beginning to understand how to approach their own problem areas. Although members will be challenged to focus this work in sessions 3 to 5, it is always valuable to mark these initial steps with encouragement. By doing so, the therapist conveys the message that efforts to implement change in their daily lives will be vital to the members' success in accomplishing the goals they have set.

The following excerpt provides an example of a member discussing his relationships. Robert begins by talking at length about his symptoms of binge eating, but notice how the therapists gently guide him away from a discussion of these symptoms to an awareness of his struggles in navigating his current relationships with his wife and father. By redirecting Robert, the therapists keep the group discussion focused on the relevant tasks at hand. At the same time, they give Robert encouragement for beginning to work on his goals by attempting to change his interactions with his wife.

> THERAPIST: Many of the goals you have created center on the important people in your lives. Much of the binge eating centers on either difficulties in relationships or lack of relationships. As people share more about how their goals are fitting for them, also talk more about these important people. Not only does it give us more information, so we understand you more fully, but it also gives us the opportunity help you in terms of achieving some of these relationship goals.
>
> ROBERT: Well, for me, last week was a pretty mellow week as far as my eating. I spent a lot of hours at work, so I didn't have a whole lot of hours to eat, which was good. I had an episode

Sunday, though. When I finished my work, I went in and started cooking, and I didn't stop until I got a phone call. Thank goodness he called me last night because I would've eaten all the way through till this morning.

CO-THERAPIST: It seemed like one of the things you shared with me, and I think a lot of you have talked about this, is that eating is a way to unwind, you know, and to kind of de-stress. Instead of talking to or doing something with someone, a friend or spouse, you'll turn to food.

ROBERT: Boy, did I unwind, right on the refrigerator. . . .

CO-THERAPIST: How are some of the other things going with working on your goals, with your relationship with your wife?

ROBERT: Good. My wife and I are actually talking quite a bit more. She's not used to that, so she's kind of wondering. But then she knows why I'm asking questions and then talking to her more, because of the group and my goals. She's pretty private herself and doesn't talk a lot, either. So it's weird for us to do that. You know it's like I try to sneak the information out of her.

CO-THERAPIST: So, that was one of the things you're working on, to share more? It is great that you are already trying to do that. I think a few others have that as a goal also.

ROBERT: Yeah, sharing with her more in general and also about how I feel about my father. He's out of the hospital. I haven't known him for very long, since we were only recently reunited, so I want to keep him around as much as I can.

NANCY: It's good to hear that he is doing better.

JEANNE: I think I told you that my daughter found me after many years—she was adopted out. . . .

This excerpt ends when Jeanne joins with Robert, by sharing a similar experience of locating her daughter after she was adopted many years ago. Most likely, if Robert had continued to discuss his symptoms, it would not have been long before the entire group joined around symptoms instead of the more productive area of the interpersonal review.

MODIFYING GOALS

Although the therapist constructs the written goals based on pre-group interviews, members may find it necessary to make some revisions. It is valuable to have members reconfigure the goals using their own words and ideas, particularly when the therapist's written goals are not clear to them or don't seem to fit, as in the following excerpt from session 2. Wendy, who has struggled with symptoms of binge eating, has been talking about her relationships—especially the one she has with her husband. When the therapist asks her later how her goals are fitting for her, she replies:

> WENDY: I completely rewrote my goals. . . . I do depend on food
> . . . when people let me down.
> THERAPIST: Is there one goal you could share with us, as a way to
> focus yourself?
> WENDY: I want to depend on my decisions, not on food. Some-
> times I will be so concerned with my husband's feelings that I
> lose my decision! In talking about our relationship, just now, I
> realize this even more.
> THERAPIST: How complex interactions become when you don't
> have clarity about how you feel. So, learning to be able to trust
> your feelings more and then take a stand for yourself is a goal
> then?
> WENDY: Yeah, with my husband. I back down too much.

As noted earlier, it is through group participation, increasing trust, and self-disclosure in the first two sessions that members begin to appreciate the complexity of their feelings and form a fuller understanding of their relationship difficulties. With encouragement, this developing insight will lead them to adjust their target goals accordingly, as the following example illustrates:

Tom is a thirty-seven-year-old married man with one child who works as a teacher. In the pregroup interviews and session 1, he described himself as happily married for nine years and glad that at least one area of his life was OK. He went on to mention that one of his target goals was to learn how to better express himself at work, where, for a second time, he had been passed over for a position he wanted. His symptoms of depression had gotten significantly worse around the time this happened. As he began to talk about his significant relationships in session 2, it occurred to him that he had been feeling increasingly uncomfortable with his wife. He had noticed that he didn't share with her the level of pain he felt about the lack of advancement at his job. As the group therapists encouraged him to continue and other members listened, he realized that he had been pulling away from her for some time now. As the self-imposed barrier eroded, he was more willing to look at this area of his life that he had previously needed to believe was "OK." He decided to make enhancing the intimacy in his marriage one of his goals.

CONTAINING AFFECT

The techniques described in Chapter 3 regarding the development of target goals identify core issues of maladaptive interpersonal functioning. The early sessions of the group are structured around this material. There is the potential for escalation of affect to a level where containment strategies may be required. The therapist needs to be tracking all members in this regard, especially through the engagement stage. Regular informal end-of-session debriefing interventions are helpful; for example, the therapist might ask "What has it been like to talk of these sensitive issues in this session?" or "How are people going to be feeling after they get home tonight and find themselves thinking of the important but difficult matters we talked about today?" The therapist can also slow down the group process if a general escalation is building: "Maybe it's time we just sat back a bit, took some deep breaths, and gave ourselves a little relaxation room."

In depression groups it is possible for several members with severe depression to establish a theme of hopelessness and futility that can demoralize the other members. Sometimes even a single dominant group member may keep the group in control by continually stating the impossibility of making changes because of symptoms such as low energy, poor concentration, and so on. A common argument in such situations is that depression is a brain disorder and therefore beyond one's control to alter. It is useful to bear in mind that repeated recitation of symptoms is likely to lead to a poor outcome. The focus on symptoms at the beginning of the group is designed to develop universality and acceptance. But after the engagement stage, symptom-focused discussions need to be dampened. Toward this end, the therapist may have to be relatively direct and firm about keeping the group on task.

THE GROUP AS SUBSTITUTE SOCIAL WORLD

As group cohesion begins to develop in these early sessions, members will find it tempting to consider the group their primary social resource. Among the major advantages of group psychotherapy are the supportive and containing properties of a cohesive group. The therapist, always in an ambivalent position, may need to regularly reinforce the importance of applying what is being discussed in the group to outside interpersonal and social connections. Helpful in this regard are informal application tasks followed by a reporting back to the group as to how well they have gone. IPT-G does not use homework assignments, so the therapist's expectations of outside application need to be clearly spelled out.

SUMMARY

The group climate intensifies in session 2 as members reveal more about themselves, their relationships, and their reactions. The group is on track if members are able to discuss key people in their lives, begin to show signs of connection to each other, and demonstrate some understanding of the association between symptoms and interpersonal functioning. Concerns in this session are usually related to members learning how to identify and manage the emotions that arise within them while they are in the group. Some will hint that they feel overwhelmed with these emotions and, depending on the symptoms that brought them to the group, may feel an urge to call off work the next day (because of depression) or binge eat later. Taking the time to do a thorough wrap-up will aid members in preparing to leave this session. Members may also be apprehensive about "fitting in" with the group or question whether the group will be helpful to them. It is useful, therefore, to urge members to stick with it, and to let them know that they will feel more comfortable as they become more trusting of each other. The main points introduced in sessions 1 and 2 establish the substructure from which the rest of the group will develop. (See Table 4.2 for a summary checklist covering session 2.)

THE END OF THE INITIAL PHASE: SESSIONS 3 TO 5

Depending on the number of group members and their ability to work together, it will take some time to thoroughly cover all of the tasks introduced in the initial phase of treatment. Sessions 3 to 5 are geared toward preparing members for the next step: the work stage. During this stage, members continue to refine their target goals; they also begin to work on them on a daily basis. The expectation is that, by session 5, the majority will have begun tackling one or two target goals.

FEEDBACK

Partly on the basis of the structure provided in the first two sessions, members will have become more invested in each other's work and their own by session 3. At this point, they will begin to appreciate the idea that to recover they need to share more in depth about themselves and the issues confronting them. Many, however, will become vigilant to the reactions of others as they strive to do this. Since members will have more knowledge about each other by this time, they

TABLE 4.2   Summary Checklist for Session 2

Therapist Tasks

1. Start and end group on time.
2. Review introductions and important structural aspects of IPT, as needed.
3. Teach members their role in IPT treatment.
4. Cultivate positive group norms:
   - Encourage all members to join discussion of interpersonal relationships related to target goals.
   - Continue to assist members in making connections among target goals, difficulties managing relationships, and associated symptoms.
   - Facilitate member self-disclosure and awareness of feelings.
   - Help members begin to modify goals and to understand how to apply them.

Individual Patient Tasks

1. Deepen feelings of connection to other members.
2. Continue to learn how to utilize group structure and process to work on target goals.
3. Review significant interpersonal relationships.
4. Continue to make connections among target goals, difficulties managing relationships, and associated symptoms.
5. Begin to share more about self and feelings.
6. Begin to modify target goals, and understand how to apply them in daily life.

will be in a better position to provide helpful and meaningful feedback. At this stage the therapist encourages members to ask for comments or reactions from other members as a way to help the others feel less isolated and to promote reality testing. For example, a member may offer words of encouragement to dispel unfounded fears that others sometimes hold about themselves:

THERAPIST: Helen, I want to check out with you because you had said something important, that you hadn't said to anyone— other than your family. Nobody knew about your son's autism and I just wondered what it was like for you to talk about that?

HELEN: I don't talk about it because I'm afraid people will say "Oh well, if he's autistic, then something must be wrong with her, too."

THERAPIST: One thing that's really important about this kind of environment is that if you ever wonder what people might be

thinking about you, this is an opportunity to ask. Because issues always come up like "Well, I'm not sure how people are
feeling toward me." We may say "Well, do you want to check
that out and ask people?"

JEANNE: Helen, you know, my husband did not meet my sister,
who also has a mental illness, until this year and I've been married twenty-one years! So I understand about the hiding because it's a very, very difficult thing to deal with mental illness
in the family.

A note of caution is offered about the term *feedback*. Therapists generally use it in a technical sense, but members may interpret it as a direction to make corrective or critical comments, or to "give advice."
Thus members should specifically be guided to provide positive
feedback, as this is a powerful tool that addresses core self-esteem issues. It is useful to establish an atmosphere in which members feel
they have a responsibility to be supportive as well as to provide constructive help with difficult issues.

WORKING ON GOALS

It may become evident to the group therapists that certain members
are experiencing difficulties related to the task of goal setting or daily
application. Some may need to continue to work at either consolidat-
ing target goals or understanding how to utilize the group format.
Others may not have become fully involved in the group. This is a serious matter because such members are at risk for dropping out.
Their perception of the group and their role in it needs to be explored.
Usually other members are able to collaborate in this effort.

Still other members may be struggling to know where to begin
their endeavors. They may have a designated problem area or two,
but with several target goals under each, and thus feel overwhelmed
about how and where to begin. The therapist may need to help these
members refine their goals and decide where to begin work. In this
situation the members can be encouraged to choose a specific goal to

start with, so they will feel less overwhelmed with change. The therapist may also recommend that members begin to take active steps, rather than waiting until "it all makes sense."

The following excerpts address three common issues that may arise in these early sessions. In the first excerpt, the therapist introduces the idea that some members may need further assistance. Samantha replies by mentioning her struggles over the question of what to do to begin work on her goals. First, to illustrate one approach to Samantha's issues, the therapist draws her attention to the way another member (Nancy) has been working. Then the therapist helps Samantha to slow down and recognize her feelings rather than rushing to take action. Finally, the therapist asks others whether they connect to this salient issue, which is common in binge eating groups:

> THERAPIST: As we prepare to start the work stage of treatment in the next few weeks, we wanted to get reactions on how goals have been fitting for each of you and how the group is going in general. Some of you have already begun to work on things, but if anyone is still unclear about their target goals, today is a good time to bring it up.
>
> SAMANTHA: I did look at my goals and even though they're overwhelming, I thought about, like, adding another one so I wrote it up. Do you want me to give it to you?
>
> THERAPIST: I'd like to see that and we can go through that a little bit. I also want to encourage you to push, like Nancy was talking about earlier, challenge yourself a little bit at those times to not binge eat and see how that works for you.
>
> SAMANTHA: I don't know what to do with whatever's going on.
>
> THERAPIST: Then part of the work for you is to really get you focusing in on what it is that's going on.
>
> SAMANTHA: Yeah, but, like, if I figure out, then what do I do with it?
>
> THERAPIST: All right. But do you know what it is that you are thinking or feeling about what is going on for you?

SAMANTHA: Sometimes, yeah. Some of my fear is, "So and so won't like this or me" and "This and this will happen," or I feel angry. Once I find it, it's like well, okay, now what? And so I don't know what to do with it, so I eat.

MARK: Eating isn't working for me like it seemed to before; does it seem to be helping you to eat over it?

SAMANTHA: Yeah, temporarily. And then, yeah, it isn't solving what is going on.

THERAPIST: So it is important for you at this point to work on focusing in on what is going on for you at those times . . . then we can move to what to do with it. Are others struggling around this same issue that Samantha is raising?

MARK: Yeah, I notice eating isn't working the same way for me, but I still don't know what to do with myself.

In the next excerpt, the group therapists have asked members to comment on their progress with goals. This example illustrates how a therapist might call attention to the ways in which a member has indeed begun to take action, even when the member is not acknowledging the successes herself. As in the previous example, the group therapist reminds Rose to take the preliminary step of examining her feelings on both sides of an issue before taking action:

ROSE: I haven't done anything in that regard, to be honest. I really haven't. And I thought about that last week because I could have gone and put myself in social situations and I frankly didn't. So I really haven't done anything.

THERAPIST: But it sounds like you have been making good connections about your level of stress and your symptoms.

ROSE: Yeah, and the other thing I have been doing on a positive note for myself is I make myself go to the gym and I feel better after I do it. And it does affect my depression level, too. I don't get as depressed when I ride that bike for an hour. I've got something coming up I'd like to talk about related to my goals:

I've been thinking about confronting my father, just actually first sort of questioning him about some things and see what he has to say. I have real fears about doing it.

THERAPIST: Well, maybe it would be important to just talk about the pros and cons.

ROSE: Yeah, it's something that I've been thinking about but I don't know what to do about it.

CAROLINE: I'm surprised to hear you say you haven't done anything, Rose; I think you've done a lot of work in such a short time. Now thinking about confronting your dad . . . I'm trying to work on speaking up more, too.

The final excerpt is taken from the third session of a group for patients with major depression. In earlier sessions Mary was an active member, almost dominating the group as members discussed depression and its effects. Notice that, in this third session, the therapist is effective in bringing in other members to address the issue raised by Mary and to assist her in thinking about taking steps toward working on this issue:

MARY: Well, this has been a week from hell. My mother called and insisted I go over and help her clean house, then my son got the flu, so I had to look after him. To top it all off my sister called and wanted me to come over and meet her new boyfriend. By Saturday, I had all I could take. So, I told my husband he would have to look after everything and I went to bed.

THERAPIST: It does sound like it has been difficult. I was thinking that you had described yourself at the beginning as not being able to set limits, and it sounds like that theme was going on this week. Carol, you had said that this was the sort of problem you often encounter. What do you make of what Mary is reporting?

CAROL: Well, I know just what she is going through. Mary, you just need to get up your courage and learn to say "no." After our meeting last week, I went home and actually told my husband he has to help out more with the kids. And, you know, he said, "OK." I almost fell over!

JOHN: I agree because you don't have trouble speaking up in here, Mary.

As illustrated in these three excerpts, members need assistance in learning how to begin to take concrete steps to work on goals. This task will become the primary focus of the intermediate sessions.

POTENTIAL NORMATIVE CHALLENGES

A few members may voice complaints about the structure and strategies of IPT at some point during the initial phase of treatment. We have found that these complaints often center on (1) the focus on current application, (2) the short-term duration, and (3) insufficient direct advice or recommendations. If the group is to move beyond these complaints to the work stage, the therapist needs to address them as they arise.

Regarding the first complaint, some members may take issue with the idea that group therapists really mean to keep the focus on current problems and relationships. For instance, several members of the same group may challenge the therapist if they have had similar difficult childhood experiences that they wish to discuss at greater length. These members can create quite a force in the group if not addressed promptly. Members may suggest that the therapists don't care enough about them as individuals if the therapists are not willing to change the format of the group to best fit the members' previous conception of group therapy. In such cases it is helpful to remind members that although the focus is on current issues, the past has, of course, influenced the way they manage their relationships in the present. To work on these problems, the therapists can examine how the old issues are perpetuated in the immediate difficulties. When members raise this issue, most of the time they are hoping to be reassured that they can mention significant past experiences in the group and that other members appreciate the difficulties that have impacted their lives.

Therapists should also anticipate criticisms about the short-term nature of the group. In larger groups, especially, members may harbor fears that their issues will not be addressed since there are so many others to attend to first. They may also feel overwhelmed about the number of goals they have set for themselves to accomplish by the group's end. The therapists can approach these matters in several ways. They can attend to each member in turn and ensure that they participate to some degree in every group. They can remind members that they have twenty weeks together to pursue their goals. And they can suggest that as the group is one step toward recovery (though not a cure for most members), they should break their work into smaller steps.

Finally, members may ask for specific recommendations, advice, or homework when working on the general goal of decreasing symptoms. For instance, it is common for members with binge eating disorder to request specific meal plans and for depressed patients to ask for a review of their medications. Although members should not be discouraged from seeking this type of information elsewhere, it is important that the therapists promptly refocus the session on current interpersonal interactions and associated goals, as this is the primary intervention strategy in IPT.

ENDING THE INITIAL PHASE

The end of the initial phase is often marked by a session in which a deeper level of affect is revealed. This change brings with it an awareness of the depth of distress that the members have been experiencing and provides a strong motivation for further work. If all group members have been participating effectively until this point, the therapist may simply acknowledge that the group seems to be ready to get on with their work. To gauge this readiness more systematically, the group therapists can check in with the members in session 5 to ensure that all have made the necessary connections between their symptoms, interpersonal problem areas, and associated target goals. The following excerpt illustrates how a therapist might wrap up this initial phase of treatment—specifically, by identifying the deepening process and reinforcing the group members' responsibility for keeping each other focused on goal areas:

> THERAPIST: Today's session seems to have really gotten into quite a bit more depth about the issues everyone has been working on. Understandably that brings with it more emotions about your situations and the challenges of addressing your goals. I wonder how it's been for each of you.
>
> TED: I felt I just had to take a deep breath and get on with it. It's been a relief to get some things off my chest.
>
> SARAH: When Joyce started to cry I really wanted to go over and hug her. But I guess she got through it by herself; good for her!
>
> JOYCE: I went into a numb state for a while, I think because I have always avoided addressing issues head-on. But I came out of it, and I'm glad I talked about that situation with my father because I know it's something that has to be resolved.
>
> THERAPIST: Well, this is hard work, but we're off to a good start. I wanted to just mark this as an important point in terms of transition for the group. This marks the end of the first phase of treatment where we've been trying to get everybody on board with your goals. Now the challenge is to keep on target with the goals everyone has. We will all struggle with that because it's understandable to want to put difficult issues on the back shelf. So everyone needs to help each other get back on track if they stray into less important areas. We're all in this together. See you all next week.

SUMMARY

The principal shift between the initial and work phases has to do with the depth of the work. In the initial stage, the goal is recognition

TABLE 4.3   Summary Checklist for Sessions 3 to 5

Therapist Tasks

---

1. Start and end group on time.
2. Ensure that members have a clear understanding of IPT rationale and roles of the therapist and members.
3. Cultivate positive group norms:
   - Maximize member self-disclosure, and heighten awareness of feeling states.
   - Keep group member discussions centered on current problem areas.
   - Continue to assist members in making connections between target goals and difficulties managing relationships.
   - Encourage members to discuss problems, changes, and successes in applying target goals.
4. Work with members who are struggling to make connections, and encourage them to note the efforts of others as a way to assist them in pushing their work forward.
5. Prepare members to enter the work stage.

Individual Patient Tasks

---

1. Deepen feelings of connection to other members.
2. Continue to learn how to utilize group structure and process to work on target goals.
3. Continue to make connections among target goals, difficulties in interpersonal relationships, and symptoms.
4. Modify target goals.
5. Begin applying target goals to daily life outside of group.
6. Share problems, changes, and successes in applying target goals.
7. Solidify goals.
8. Discuss feelings regarding the end of the initial phase.

---

of important problem areas and associated target goals that need to be addressed. The group is prepared to move on to the work stage if members have a clear understanding of their goals and have begun to take a productive role in the sessions by bringing in relevant material regarding successes and difficulties in daily application. As members will pace themselves differently, the therapist's techniques need to be adjusted accordingly. For instance, some members may be starting to apply goals and thus will need encouragement to continue their efforts, whereas others may still be struggling to self-disclose. As the group moves into the work stage, the expectation of exploration and outside application will increase. As a result, the level of affect in the group will also increase, creating opportunities for challenges between the therapist and the group as well as among the members themselves. (See Table 4.3 for a summary checklist covering sessions 3 to 5.)

CHAPTER 5

The Intermediate Phase

The intermediate phase of treatment begins after the members have clearly defined their problem areas in the group and firmly set the treatment contract in sessions 1 to 5. The bulk of the work on problem areas will occur during this phase. The therapist introduces the IPT strategies specific to each problem area to help members reach their goals. The strategies can be introduced in the context of the ongoing group discussion whenever appropriate, but they should be specifically outlined. The therapist promotes the work of the intermediate phase by keeping the group on task, which involves guiding members to:

- maintain a focus on discussing issues related to their problem areas;
- maximize self-disclosure;
- connect to and learn from other group members;
- express their emotional reactions primarily in relation to addressing their target goals and interacting with the therapist and with other members;
- implement changes based on problem areas in outside circumstances and in the group; and
- remain motivated to continue in treatment.

It is now expected that the level of discussion will move to deeper exploration of the issues that each member identified during the engagement stage as being central to recovery. Members will begin to take on more responsibility for the direction and course of the group in the intermediate phase, whereas the therapist will increasingly function as a facilitator. The rules and norms of the group will begin to consolidate and to become more clearly understood by all group members. With guidance from the therapist, members will increasingly attend to affective states, starting with outside past experiences and eventually addressing affect experienced in the group sessions.

Members will also become more comfortable with self-disclosure and learn to better give and receive profitable feedback during this "work" stage. A significant turning point can occur early when group members become more willing to openly disagree with one another. As conflict is effectively managed in this phase, the group will become increasingly concerned with building intermember harmony and cohesiveness.

The intensity of interaction that arises during this phase can foster positive feelings and a sense of fraternity. As the members contribute individually to the group atmosphere and develop a sense of "belonging," they begin to feel that they are part of an environment that facilitates change. When one member makes changes, others often report a sense of moving forward as well. Seeing others take small steps toward goals can prove synergistic to others, especially those who are having trouble getting started. Seeing that any step will be met with encouragement does much to provide the momentum that is needed during the "work" stage of IPT-G.

The specific strategies used by the therapist to facilitate the work of the intermediate phase will be based on the particular problem areas that members bring to the group. In the following sections, the four primary problem areas are reviewed and goals and intervention strategies are outlined, followed by case examples illustrating how a member works within the group format in each of the problem areas specified.

GRIEF

Goals: (1) Facilitate the mourning process. (2) Help the patient re-establish interest and relationships to substitute what has been lost.

Strategies: (1) Reconstruct the patient's relationship with the deceased. (2) Describe the sequence and consequences of events just prior to, during, and after the death. (3) Explore associated feelings (negative and positive). (4) Help the patient consider ways of becoming reinvolved with others.

The grief problem area in IPT is restricted to situations involving death. Grief is a universal reaction to the death of a person to whom one has been meaningfully connected. It is experienced as a unique form of loss. Sadness and depression may be found in other contexts of loss, but these are dealt with under another problem area. Although normal bereavement has many of the features of depression, it gradually resolves over a period of several months through social support and does not require psychiatric treatment. A return to previous levels of social and work functioning is anticipated. IPT is designed as an effective treatment for an abnormal or delayed grief reaction in which the various phases of the normal mourning process have not occurred.

An abnormal grief reaction may occur immediately following the loss or at a later time when some event or situation serves as a reminder of the loss, sometimes in the form of an "anniversary reaction." This reaction commonly takes the form of a major depression in which the connections to the bereavement may not be immediately evident. Nonspecific physical symptoms may further complicate the diagnostic task. For that reason, the assessment of a depressed state should always include a careful history concerning the deaths of important significant others. This history should include the circumstances of the death as well as the patient's emotional and behavioral reaction to it. Most abnormal grief reactions are related to difficulties

TABLE 5.1   Major Features of an Abnormal Grief Reaction

1. Reaction to multiple losses
2. Evidence of missing or inadequate grief in the bereavement period
3. Avoidance behavior about the death
4. Symptoms occurring around the anniversary of the death
5. Fear of the illness that caused the death
6. Preservation of the deceased's environment as a "shrine"
7. Reaction to absence of family or social supports during the bereavement period
8. Intrusive thoughts and memories concerning the deceased beyond the usual mourning period

in the preceding relationship with the deceased or to deaths that occurred in an unusual or untimely manner. Table 5.1 lists the major features of an abnormal grief reaction.

TREATMENT OF ABNORMAL GRIEF

The management of abnormal grief reactions is perhaps theoretically the most straightforward of the four problem areas. When memories and thoughts about the deceased person are stimulated, the grieving process is rekindled. A particularly important objective is to determine the specific details of the events prior, during, and after the death. Associated feelings should also be explored. (Certain themes may complicate this working-through process; these are listed in Table 5.2.) For the patient this is often a difficult and painful experience, to which the group members and the therapist are not immune. However, a cohesive group can be a powerful support for a member working through grief issues. The group can provide validation for the feelings being addressed and question unrealistic ideas or distortions that may accompany the disclosure of details of the event. The therapist must be prepared to assist the group members in helping the member to stick with this task. It is not uncommon for a major portion of a group session to be devoted to the initial opening up of grief issues.

The group acts as a substitute social network that may not have been available at the time of death. The diversity of grief experiences

TABLE 5.2   Typical Themes in Grief Work

1. Fear of the effects of addressing the death or even thinking about it, particularly that they will not be able to contain themselves in the process
2. Shame at not being able to prevent or postpone the event
3. Rage at others involved in the event
4. Guilt or shame over destructive fantasies about the event or those involved
5. Survivor guilt over the fact that the deceased is gone and they are still here but "deserve" to have died
6. Fear of identification or merging with the deceased
7. Overpowering sadness at the loss that seems insurmountable

among the members of a typical group provides a rich source of consolation, reassurance, and corrective reorientation: "I know just what you were experiencing, I thought I'd never get over it, but I finally did and found some peace about the whole situation. Just keep at it." A group can provide such genuinely constructive comments with great expertise. The therapist may be able to remain quite inactive throughout this process, merely monitoring the group to ensure that it stays on task and does not push any member too hard or too fast. Indeed, the most important work is probably done by the group members themselves, as many of them will be able to identify as equals in this universal human dilemma.

The next stage of the process is to reconstruct the nature of the relationship with the deceased. This more challenging task is one in which the therapist may need to take a more active role. The goal is a factual and emotionally focused understanding of the relationship, which, after the initial cathartic opening, may be set up by the therapist with the suggestion that it would be helpful for each member to take time to think more about the relationship—in terms of both its good aspects and its more stressful aspects. This outside work must then be followed up in the next session. The group may be particularly interested in the negative side of the relationship, seeing it, perhaps correctly, as a component of the abnormal grief. At this point the therapist may need to function as a rate controller to maintain the affect level of each member within a workable range. Presenting this as a task for the group as well may be helpful. And asking the group members to reflect on their own mixed feelings about losses may provide a normalizing effect.

Action-oriented techniques can also be introduced. Visiting the grave may be recommended, along with the instruction to stay for some time and perhaps speak to the deceased. Writing letters to the deceased that can be read aloud to the group may help the members bring about affect release and develop a deeper understanding regarding the complexity of the relationship. The goal would be to develop a more balanced view of the deceased.

Finally, it is important to guide the members toward new involvement with others. Joining and participating in the group itself can be seen as a first step. In addition, the members can be encouraged to think about ways to become more involved with others again in their daily lives (by dating, joining organizations, and so on).

The techniques listed here are similar to those used in the individual treatment of abnormal grief reactions. However, the group environment offers additional depth and the opportunity for normalizing the process. Since death is a universal experience, the group can usually address the related issues with an immediate understanding that is less easily achieved in the other problem areas. At the same time, the group itself is conducive to a socialization process that can serve as a model for application in outside relationships.

THE CASE OF HARRY

Initial phase (sessions 1 to 5): Harry, a forty-five-year-old widower, was assessed as having an abnormal grief reaction concerning the death of his wife five years earlier, with chronic symptoms of major depression since then. This situation had seriously impacted his ability to work at a middle management position, and his vocational status had slowly dropped. His wife had had a chronic illness for several years and he had assumed the main responsibility for their three young children. Throughout the marriage his wife had been highly critical and often made demeaning remarks about him in public. He suffered this in silence and deferred to her demands. These patterns escalated as her physical condition deteriorated. He experienced enormous guilt at her death because of the sense of relief he experienced with her demise. He had continuing intrusive thoughts about both the excitement and romance of their early years and the anger during the later stages. In early sessions, Harry was a very helpful and empathic group member, well liked by the group. Despite invitations to address his situation, he never got beyond a simple statement of how hard it had been. The other group members were perhaps reluctant to have their supportive member change roles.

Intermediate phase (sessions 6 to 15): As the group was approaching the one-third point, the therapist basically said it was time and encouraged the group to assist in helping Harry address his difficult task. With much hesitation and the group's gentle urging his story began to come out, and with it several periods of deep sobs. Harry then spoke of his sense of shame at "breaking down" and revealing family secrets. Two group members spoke of similar reactions to losses. At the end of the session, the therapist reviewed how Harry felt about the session, and he replied that it had been enormously helpful, though frightening too. He was encouraged to continue his grief work with his one close friend and to report back at the next session. Over several additional sessions, more aspects of his marriage came out and Harry's mood became significantly more elevated. He brought in his wedding picture and passed it around the room.

Termination phase (sessions 16 to 20): Toward the end of the group, Harry reported a sense of a great weight having been lifted and he thought he might be able to get on with his life again. With some embarrassment he reported at the second to last session that he had had a date. The group was of course delighted.

This case illustrates how the therapist increasingly raised the expectation of dealing with a central issue that had been identified in the assessment procedure. Once the material was opened, much of the actual therapeutic work was conducted between Harry and the group members.

The therapist should strive for therapy through the group process. At the same time, other group members will have burning issues to explore. Since grief is such a common human experience, there may be a tendency to stick with this material as a less controversial area. The therapist must be prepared to titrate the available time to prevent such a development. However, observing a grief reaction improve may provide a positive model for other group members to imitate in their own problem area.

INTERPERSONAL ROLE DISPUTES

Goals: (1) Identify the dispute. (2) Help the patient choose a plan of action. (3) Modify the patient's expectations or faulty communications to bring about a satisfactory resolution.

Strategies: (1) Determine the stage of the dispute: renegotiation (calm down participants to facilitate resolution); impasse (increase disharmony in order to reopen negotiation); or dissolution (assist mourning and adaptation). (2) Understand how nonreciprocal role expectations relate to the dispute: What are the issues in the dispute? What are the differences in expectations and values? What are the options? What is the likelihood of finding alternatives? What resources are available to bring about change in the relationship? Are there parallels in other relationships? What is the patient gaining? What unspoken assumptions lie behind the patient's behavior? How is the dispute perpetuated?

Interpersonal role disputes (RDs) occur when the group member and a significant other have contradictory role expectations about their relationship. These nonreciprocal expectations are usually being managed either covertly as stony silences or overtly as arguments. Role dispute issues can be revealed in what a member both says and doesn't say. For example, a member may provide either an overly idealized description or scanty information about an important other. Both depictions should be investigated further for the possibility of RD issues. Factors that perpetuate role disputes are the member's belief that nothing can be done, poor communication strategies, and irreconcilable differences. In most instances of RD, members are concerned that they have no control over the dispute; some may fear the total loss of the relationship.

Interpersonal role disputes are probably the most common category of issues found in situations of psychological distress. Role disputes are also frequently cited as a secondary problem area. (In one case, for example, a woman struggling with an unresolved grief reaction lost an important resource because her intense need for support eventually alienated her closest friend.) The strategies for dealing with role disputes may be helpful in such situations once the primary problem area begins to be better managed.

TREATMENT OF INTERPERSONAL ROLE DISPUTES

The first task in the RD problem area is to assess the status of the role dispute in terms of renegotiation, impasse, or dissolution. Although this assessment begins in the pregroup meetings, the initial-phase sessions offer an opportunity for further exploration of the issue before a final direction is chosen. If the dispute is at the *renegotiation* stage, there is still a sense of engagement between the individuals involved—even if they have been unsuccessful in bringing about changes. If so, the focus would move immediately toward clarifying the basis of the misunderstanding, thus emphasizing the nature of the reciprocal roles between enacted. It may emerge that tension in the relationship has been stuck at an *impasse* for some time, accompanied by distancing remoteness or unremitting antagonism. A role dispute at such an impasse will need to be activated in order to move into a workable direction (i.e., either renegotiation or dissolution), thus inevitably increasing the level of anxiety and tension in the involved relationship.

Alternatively, it may be that resolution by moving into renegotiation is not possible or is not the best choice of action. In this instance, the focus may shift to *dissolution* of the relationship. This decision is likely to bring a sense of relief and an opening of opportunities, but also regrets. The strategies used will be similar to those in the grief problem area. It may involve, first, a closer look at what is being given up and, then, an examination of what transition tasks must be addressed. Emotional reactions to the changes must also be accounted for.

The therapist will need to monitor these exploratory discussions carefully, making sure to stop early advice-giving in the group. Other group members may seize upon an alternative stance and exert pressure for an early decision, which may take the general form of "You would be better of without that jerk/witch." Such responses, based as they are on limited knowledge, may ignore underlying remediable opportunities or the high degree of ambivalence that the patient is masking. It is not the task of other group members or the therapists to determine the course of action to be taken. That remains the individual group member's decision. The initial public disclosure of the problematic situation in the group and the relief associated with affective ventilation frequently promote serious reflection on the nature of the dispute. The question of change becomes more real, going beyond mere hypothetical imagining. Impulsive decisions should be avoided.

The early focus on the RD process is intended to clarify nonreciprocal role expectations. Thus it often involves an examination of unclear communications between the protagonists and requires that the basis of underlying issues be probed. Differences in expectations or values may be revealed. For example, the relationship may not be meeting poorly understood wishes for support, control, or intimacy. It is most helpful if similar patterns in previous relationships or in current group interactions can be found. By encouraging exploration of the emotional tension being experienced by the patient in the group and its direct connections to the outside dispute, the therapist can relieve some of the pressure and allow a more objective view of the situation. As an example, consider the following case:

> Jane spoke at length in early sessions about how controlling her husband
> was and about the absence of love in their marriage. Several women in the

group echoed this theme and pressed Jane to initiate a discussion of separation. The therapist cautioned direct advice and encouraged a deeper look at the relationship. This led to the further revelation, as the group progressed, that her husband provided the major share of child-rearing responsibilities and that Jane was continually berating him for his failings, which she viewed as the major trigger for her bingeing/purging episodes. Gradually the group's attitude changed and the members were able to address the high level of control that Jane herself appeared to exert in the home and, indeed, how her initial presentation quite dominated the group interaction, leading to some resentment by other members at not getting their fair share of time. This discussion triggered a helpful process for Jane in beginning to address the role imbalance at home. Note that most of this work was done by group members with subtle prompting by the therapist.

The development of a cohesive and interactive group will provide both a model and a platform upon which to practice more effective dispute resolution. This atmosphere promotes a new and expanded look at personal problems in relationships. Difficulties in addressing the need to confront and not tolerate negative feelings may be resulting in an avoidance of efforts to achieve a solution. The therapist can assist this process by regularly encouraging members to describe how they are responding to the issues being raised. It is most important that the therapist model a direct, open, and nonconfrontational approach to the core issues of all members. In order for the group to move on toward addressing solutions, the process of clarification and identification of these issues must begin early.

THE CASE OF MARJORIE

Marjorie is a thirty-seven-year-old middle manager. She has risen steadily in her demanding job, and much of her self-worth is invested in it. She travels frequently and often works overtime. She emigrated from abroad in her early twenties, primarily to get away from her mother, whom she describes as intensely intrusive, critical, and filled with advice. She harbors strong feelings of resentment over the fact that her mother always treats her like a child and never validates her opinions and actions. These feelings appear to have kept her closely tied to her mother, and she wonders whether they are connected to her difficulty in forgiving her mother for the past. Even her geographic move has not resolved this situation; for the past fifteen years she has talked with her mother at least once per week. Each of these conversations leaves her seething, but she has not been able to decrease their frequency.

Marjorie had several relationships with men when she was in her twenties, each lasting for a couple of years. From these men she received companionship but never expressions of deeper commitment. In each case, the man initiated separation, and on each occasion she felt devastated; on two such occasions she suffered a major depressive episode. She describes an intense need to find another partner immediately. She has a small circle of girlfriends whom she sees sporadically.

Initial phase (sessions 1 to 5): Marjorie describes her current depression as being directly connected to her six-year relationship with a man in a similar occupation, with whom she has regular contact around business matters. Some twelve years her senior, he is married and has no intention of ending his marriage, though she describes the marriage as loveless. Fearing business gossip, they have conducted a clandestine relationship in out-of-the-way hotels, restaurants, and vacation retreats.

In early group sessions, Marjorie was direct and verbal regarding these matters, showing little overt emotion. She was clear that she loved this man, yet also felt quite ambivalent about the future of the relationship. On the one hand, she feared it would not progress from its present state into a full and committed union. On the other, she found herself quite dependent on the relationship to fulfill legitimate emotional needs for a close bond with someone. She stated that this impasse strongly affected her feelings about herself and her future. One major component of these feelings was her desire to have children and his adamant refusal to even consider the possibility.

Marjorie had three primary issues at the start of the initial phase. One was to resolve this intimate relationship, which she clearly recognized as being at an impasse. She also wanted to address her relationship with her mother—in particular, the distress she experienced after each telephone conversation. Finally, she felt that she should expand the frequency of her contacts with friends, which had diminished as she became more depressed.

She emerged as a strong and helpful member early in the group. The other members seemed puzzled at the contrast between her assured competency and her difficulty in resolving the relationship with her lover. She received much advice about getting out of the situation by ending it. The therapist repeatedly intervened to caution others about making decisions for her and encouraged them to try to understand both sides of the situation. Another woman in the group had experienced a similar situation and was able to align with Marjorie's underlying yearning for a supportive and loving relationship. This exchange provided an opportunity for a major cathartic disclosure of Marjorie's sense of isolation and weakness in managing this relationship.

At this point, Marjorie's role in the group shifted and she became another member rather than a co-therapist. In a sense, she removed her business competency and could then look at her interpersonal vulnerability. By the end of the initial phase, although her target goals remained the same, she had decided that the only suitable course would be to move toward dissolution of the relationship. This decision did not seem to be impulsive; rather, it was intended to bring to a head the direction she was previously fearful of taking.

Intermediate phase (sessions 6 to 15): Marjorie delved into the issue rapidly. She challenged her lover again about having children, and again he was opposed. It appeared that the forcefulness of her request surprised him and he became somewhat distant. Her fears of losing him were reactivated. Throughout the first four weeks of the intermediate phase, this process occurred several times. Each time, the group provided support and a realistic reflection of the situation. Two other women were addressing somewhat similar problems in their intimate relationships, and it was very helpful for Marjorie to see their struggles. Her own doubts and fears were normalized, making them less intense. At the formal midpoint review of target goals in the group, Marjorie was able to state that she was ready to end the relationship and proceeded to do so. The nature of her business connections with her lover became exceedingly formal. She reestablished her connections with several friends and organized a vacation with one of them.

Marjorie continued to mourn the loss of the relationship during the later intermediate phase. But having followed through on her decision, she was now freed up to address the tensions with her mother. She had several forthright conversations with her mother around her critical comments and set limits on the frequency and duration of their phone calls. She seemed better able to see her mother as an aging woman whose "style" was not likely to change. This realization made it easier to tolerate her mother's language without experiencing the previous degree of rage.

Termination phase (sessions 16 to 20): The group entered the termination phase by discussing the theme of losses, and several members spoke of earlier deaths and the impact they had had on their lives. In the course of these discussions, Marjorie burst into tears. Between sobs, she recounted an abortion she had at an early age. Feeling that she could not tell her mother about this, she had managed the entire experience without support. It was at this time that she determined to leave her home country for good. She also spoke of this event as driving her current desire to have a child before it was too late. Several members reported parallel early experiences in the context of efforts to come to terms with old losses or injuries. The group had an emotional final session in which the importance of group understanding and support was underlined.

Marjorie in effect addressed two situations of interpersonal impasse. The first was the obvious one regarding her lover—a situation that she resolved by ending it. The second was her relationship with her mother, which she addressed by altering her internal perception of her mother, thereby detoxifying their phone calls. In addition, she addressed a grief reaction that she had harbored as a shameful secret for over twenty years.

ROLE TRANSITIONS

Goals: (1) Help the patient to mourn and accept the loss of the old role. (2) Help the patient to regard the new role as more positive. (3) Help the patient to restore self-esteem by developing a sense of mastery regarding demands of new roles.

Strategies: (1) Review positive and negative aspects of old and new roles. (2) Explore feelings about what is lost. (3) Explore feelings about the change itself. (4) Explore opportunities that the new role brings. (5) Realistically evaluate what is lost. (6) Encourage appropriate release of affect. (7) Encourage development of a social support system and of any new skills called for in the new role.

Symptoms of depression or binge eating may emerge when a life change involves assuming new roles. All people can be described as playing several roles at any point in time; however, difficulties may occur when individuals are called upon to change roles rapidly or to leave a role that they have found important to their sense of self. Taking a new job, moving, starting school, retiring, and divorcing are all examples of role transition. Some individuals are more vulnerable than others to the stresses that such changes entail. Often, people with depression experience the changes as a loss, whereas those with binge eating difficulties use food to soothe the dysphoric affect. The transition may lead some to feel a sense of failure as they struggle to adjust to the new role and the possible change in status that it brings. Loss of familiar supports, difficulty managing emotions, lower self-esteem, and a need for new social skills are some of the issues that arise during role transitions.

The therapist can also look for problems related to role transitions at those times in the life cycle when such normative transitions are a necessary part of moving through life. For example, late adolescence and early adulthood present the challenge of developing intimate relationships outside of one's family of origin and assuming a productive role in society. In middle adulthood, career and family issues come to the fore. And as one continues to age, issues of health and loss of friends through death become important changes to manage.

Role Transition Treatment

The group provides the social support system that members with role transition (RT) problem areas are often currently lacking or underutilizing. By joining this new group system, members take a first step toward addressing an important aspect of RT treatment: finding and connecting to new supports. Having a place in which to discuss recent role changes will help members to express the associated affect that may be experienced as overwhelming and conflicted when alone. Since change is a universal experience, many will identify with RT issues and be able to offer empathy and support to members with RT problem areas.

As members with RT issues become more comfortable in the group, they can be led to examine both positive and negative aspects of their old and new roles. Feedback from group members can be productive when members with RT problem areas begin to glorify the old roles while disregarding the benefits of the new ones. For instance, a forty-year-old man moved to take a job that was better suited to him, but he had difficulty adapting to small-town life. He idealized his old job and friends, and group members were effective in giving him feedback about his tendency to do this. Eventually he came to realize that, because he was uncomfortable in his new role, he had been suppressing his memory of the extent to which he and his old boss did not get along and the negative consequences it had on his work environment.

The therapist specifically needs to encourage expression of affect around the changes that have been required when a patient leaves an old role and assumes a new role. Feelings of disappointment may arise if the old role was one that the patient attempted but did not succeed in. Feelings of emptiness may occur if the old role was part of a phase of life that is now over, such as children leaving home. Every group member has been through these types of changes and will have something to offer by way of common experience.

By merely interacting with others in the group, members with RT problem areas can reacquaint themselves with important social skills they have used in the past to connect with others but may have stopped using. They can also gain insight into the feelings and beliefs that are blocking them from using their skills outside by noticing their hesitation to connect with others in the group. Learning to use these skills again or developing new ones will provide a sense of mastery.

Transitions often require a change in social supports. Joining the group is one way to break the cycle of isolation among individuals who have bypassed opportunities for social contact while attempting to cope with the stresses of role change. Reaching out to others may help to ease such transitions, but it also means that they must risk getting to know new people at a time when they already feel vulnerable. Group members can provide support and encourage those with RT problem areas to connect with others in their social environment.

THE CASE OF WW

WW is a fifty-one-year-old woman who is college educated and a divorced mother of one adult son in his early twenties. WW began binge eating at age fourteen. At one point she developed a dependence on diet pills; she also had one past episode of major depression. When she presented to treatment for binge eating, her weight was 205 pounds, above the 95th percentile. She had previous episodes of binge eating related to a move to a new location and had sought individual counseling. She presented to group treatment when her symptoms worsened after she moved recently from another country to the United States. She had not been able to form new social supports. Before the move, her son had gone back to live with his father, a development that was very troublesome to her.

WW describes herself as a "social person," and she comes across that way to those who meet her. She carries herself with confidence and works hard to been seen as competent. However, living in a new country and being alone in the evenings and on weekends have raised feelings of loneliness, sadness, and boredom, which in turn have precipitated the recurrence of her binge eating symptoms.

Initial phase (sessions 1 to 5): WW clearly recognized that her binge eating symptoms increased when she moved to the United States and experienced severe social isolation. Previously, she had her son with her for some company, but she has been alone since his move a year and a half ago. His move made the transition to a new country even more difficult for WW. She also said that she was starting out again, alone, "at an age that made it more difficult to make friends." Although she continued to become involved in many activities ("I'm a member of anything I can become a member of"), she said that she felt she was always doing things alone. WW clearly saw herself as out of the loop. At fifty-one, she imagined that most people at her stage in life either had lives that were "too busy" for her or already had established friends. Already feeling rejected by her son, she was quick to interpret her isolated circumstance as another rejection by the new environment. WW did point out cultural differences in the social area, saying that people in the United States "close themselves inside, nobody has time." In her previous culture, she added, there was "always time for socializing, so that you are not alone."

Based on information gathered in the pretreatment interviews and the first few sessions, the therapist decided that the group would help WW manage the role transition involved in adjusting to a new country and adapting to her adult son's decision to relocate to his father's home. Two of WW's goals were to become more aware of her emotions and to understand how binge eating seemed to be the way to manage them. She was also encouraged to think and talk about the changes brought about by the move, including the cultural adjustments. She needed to take steps to increase her social contacts in the new environment. A third goal for WW centered on the way she interacted with significant others by caretaking, even at the risk of overextending herself to make others' lives perfect. All this work on others' behalf would leave her feeling resentful and stressed, since she wasn't taking care of her own needs in the process. She needed to begin to find ways to take care of herself other than by using food.

WW participated actively in the first session and had many positive interactions with other members. A group member pointed out that she came across as "confident" and easy to talk to. One of the important insights that emerged for WW in the early sessions was that those close to her might not know that she has needs or that she feels disconnected from others. Before session 2, WW disclosed some of her feelings of isolation to her sister-in-law, who responded by increasing her efforts to spend time with WW. The group members were excited to see someone in the group risk openness and get a positive response.

In sessions 4 and 5, WW began talking more in the group about her relationship with her son. As group members heard more details and witnessed the way that WW spoke about the relationship, they began to suggest that she might have an excessively caretaking interpersonal style. This feedback and the support from other group members led her to look more directly at this aspect of her relationships, especially in terms of her son.

Intermediate phase (sessions 6 to 15): During this phase WW began to focus her work more intensely on her goals, making good progress in all areas. Intense interactions occurred at times between WW and another group member who was also struggling with issues involving her adult son. (The latter's son had a mental illness.) Whereas WW's style with her son was quite solicitous, the other members' style was one of "tough love" and placing limits. These two styles represented opposite ends of the spectrum. Both members received important reflections from each other and the group about their common interpersonal issue. As a result, both members were eventually able to change their style of interacting with their sons. For WW, this meant holding herself back from excessive caretaking. Now, instead of trying to make things perfect for him when he visited, during which he only criticized, she found ways to make sure that she attended to her own activities. She noticed that her son treated her with more respect as she made changes in her interpersonal behavior.

By placing appropriate limits in her relationship with her adult son, and recognizing his adult-like responses in return, she was freed up to see more clearly the need to evaluate her own life and where she wanted to go. Her primary role as "mom" had changed and she needed to define herself in other ways. She had been accustomed to socializing with other moms and had felt easily connected to others in this role. But now that her son had moved out and was growing into a young man, and now that she herself was living in a new country, it was time to deal with this important normative transition.

In sessions 10 to 13, WW reported significant work in initiating and establishing relationships with others. This work appeared to give her confidence in her new roles. In fact, she had begun to receive a few social invitations. She was also more attuned to the ways that she relied on food, especially when she was lonely or felt that she wasn't receiving enough time from others. The connection between the lack of supportive contacts and the binge eating was becoming very clear to her in these intermediate sessions.

Termination phase (sessions 16 to 20): In session 16, WW said that she was aware of no longer feeling so lonely and isolated and that her binge eating had decreased significantly. Then, in later sessions, she talked about her awareness of needing to let go of the past and to accept her life as it was now. This meant assuming her new roles more fully:

WW: One of the problems in my life is that I was living too much in the past with my relations, with the way I used to live with people. I've realized that there are things now and ahead to be gained, and I can't continue to always look back because then I have no opportunity to look in the present. I said to myself, "I have good friends back there, but I have nothing here." But the reality is that I don't live back there, I live here. I started to cultivate and do things here. And not looking back and saying "back there" was great, but it doesn't exist any more.

Initially, WW had thought she needed another activity to replace the binge eating, such as cross-stitching. As she became more aware of the connection between her loneliness and food and, subsequently, made efforts to establish contact with others, she pointed out that "now I don't feel that need to have an activity."

As she reviewed her progress in the group she was pleased to have established a supportive friendship network. She was also proud of herself for learning to be clear about her feelings and taking care of herself. In the future WW needs to continue to be mindful of her feelings and to balance care for others and herself. Below is an excerpt from the last session:

> WW: Many of the things that people said to me here were very important for me. Because I had nobody, the eating took over everything for me. And what can I say, I'm thrilled to see my son, I'm making new relationships, and new friends. I was a little afraid in the beginning but it has changed my life. I no longer reward myself with an ice cream sundae. Everybody here put in something to make me feel better.

INTERPERSONAL DEFICITS

Goals: (1) Reduce the patient's social isolation. (2) Encourage formation of new relationships.

Strategies: (1) Review the patient's past significant relationships, including negative and positive aspects. (2) Explore the repetitive patterns in these relationships. (3) Discuss the patient's positive and negative reactions toward both the therapists and the group members, and seek parallels in other relationships.

Individuals are diagnosed with the problem area of interpersonal deficits (IDs) when they have a history of profound and persistent disturbances in social relationships. Many of these difficulties are long-standing, leading to a failure to develop intimate adult relationships. Such individuals may lack social skills or have pervasive, maladaptive ways of reacting to relationships that prohibit their social and emotional development. Often they are quite socially isolated or involved in such a superficial manner that their relationships are chronically unfulfilling. The relationships themselves are often typified by absence of emotional expression, avoidance of conflict, fear of rejection, and lack of perceived support. Symptoms of depression or binge eating may arise from these difficulties. In this event, the therapist's strategy is to help the group member focus on the appropriate interpersonal difficulties and devise successful strategies for navigating them.

INTERPERSONAL DEFICITS TREATMENT

Participation in the group itself is a first step toward reducing isolation and increasing motivation to form new relationships, which in turn comprise the primary goal for this problem area. Since the main issue in ID is the presence of long-standing and repeated relationship difficulties that are more severe than the typical role dispute, it is inevitable that members with ID will experience strong mixed emotions as they attempt to find their place among the other group members. Others in the group will usually be able to identify with these difficulties, especially the loneliness and fear of rejection that are common among members with ID. This sense of common issues with other members may be important in allowing those with ID to reveal their relationship difficulties more readily.

The first strategy is to encourage a review of past and current relationships with the aim of discovering the social behaviors that contribute to interpersonal failures. The maladaptive ways of relating to others will become "real" as members with ID demonstrate these same behaviors in the group setting. The IPT group is an ideal forum for identifying "in vivo" these social difficulties. Encouraging an open discussion about the feelings and thoughts that the patient may have regarding others in the group, the therapist, or the therapy itself is necessary if members are to learn to negotiate relationships more effectively.

Members with ID problem areas will typically prefer to sever a relationship rather than confront others and resolve issues. For instance, members with ID as a problem area may telephone the group therapist after an intense session and say they will not return due to some distorted or unrealistic negative interpretation of what occurred in the group. The group therapist can assist interpersonal learning by encouraging these members to bring their reactions back to the group. It is important for the therapist to be ready to structure the ensuing interaction in such a way as to facilitate interpersonal learning. The experience of being guided through the process of confronting and clarifying their feelings toward the issues raised or other group members can be very helpful to ID members. It provides them with a language to understand their interpersonal relationships more clearly. Encouraging the members to notice parallels in other relationships yields fruitful insights that can lead to behavior change. These supportive interventions may help to retain an ID member who is considering terminating prematurely.

Other members, though they do not seek to sever their relationship with the group, nevertheless habitually withdraw when they are upset. These individuals may be unaware of the negative consequences of closing off communication and retreat because they feel unable to resolve difficulties in relationships. Identifying the negative aspects of this type of communication is important. The therapist can encourage the members to let others know when they are beginning to feel shut down. Becoming aware of "closing off," and being open to looking at how and when it occurs, will begin to help break the dysfunctional communication pattern.

Linking this type of interpersonal information from in-session to out-of-session interpersonal behavior is an immediate and concrete way to enhance interpersonal learning. Thus, members with ID are encouraged to develop congruent relationships within the group with therapists and members as a model for developing outside relationships.

THE CASE OF BARB

Barb is a fifty-three-year-old cosmetologist who has two adult daughters. Barb began bingeing at age fifteen and continued to diet and experience weight fluctuations for years. At the time of her initial evaluation she was having three binge episodes a week. She said she was most likely to binge when she felt uneasy. At 231 pounds she was severely overweight and at the 95th percentile for weight. She also met criteria for obsessive-compulsive personality disorder with a sub-threshold diagnosis of self-defeating personality disorder.

Barb had a history of conflict avoidance and a fear of criticism. At the age of sixteen, she began a series of failed relationships that she attempted to hide or glorify (by saying she was married when she wasn't) in order to appear as the "perfect" daughter. Accordingly, she used food to "numb out" and manage the feelings she kept private. Her attempts at secrecy and use of food to disconnect from her feelings continued throughout her first marriage. Although she reported that her husband had been cruel and verbally abusive, she "fooled everyone for eighteen years" into believing she had a fulfilling relationship, so as to hide her sense of failure.

Initial phase (sessions 1 to 5): Like all members in early group sessions, Barb was encouraged to talk about significant relationships. Since her divorce, Barb has been involved in a live-in relationship that was characterized by emotional disconnection. She hid her eating symptoms from her boyfriend, ate little when they were together, and binged later. At work, she was headed for burnout as a result of being unable to set limits with clients who demanded to be seen either before or after her regular work hours. She often found herself eating on her way home from work as a way to manage her conflicted feelings about her workload.

Instead of sharing this information with the group, Barb insisted that her relationships were wonderful and that she had no problems to speak of, other than her inability to diet effectively. Consistent with the problem area of interpersonal deficits, Barb had a hard time allowing herself to connect to others by revealing herself more honestly, thus exacerbating her distance from others. Years of lying to important people in her life and deceiving herself to maintain an image of perfection had led to Barb's inability to communicate effectively or manage conflict. Her interpersonal communication in the group took the form of apologies, and she insisted that she did not know why she was in the group because she did not have problems the others seemed to have. Other members of the group visibly bristled when she reported having had a perfect childhood and expressed sadness for group members who had it much harder than she.

A significant turning point came when other group members began to discuss their own unfulfilling relationships. Barb's fellow group members began to confront her about her claims of having such wonderful past and present relationships. In essence, they challenged her by presenting the notion that if she had problems with binge eating, her life could not be all that "together." Through this modeling and confrontation by others, along with a subsequent dialog, Barb revealed that her relationships had not been as intimate or as satisfying as she had at first suggested. This review of significant relationships and their positive and negative aspects is an important component of helping the member with an ID problem area. Although Barb began to be more accepted by other members after this interaction, her style of masking issues and holding herself as "better" continued to be a concern well into the intermediate phase of treatment.

By the end of the initial phase, the therapist decided that the group would help Barb to address her problem area by encouraging her to begin to share her feelings with others. This work would not only help to relieve the pressure that comes from holding feelings inside but also increase her connection to others, both within the group and in her outside relationships. In addition, it would involve examining her intense fear and avoidance of conflict and finding a way to better negotiate with others. Barb would also need to learn to examine her feelings so as to identify them instead of using food to manage.

Throughout the rest of the initial phase, Barb began addressing her goal of taking care of herself and sharing more with her boyfriend. As a result of reducing her workload and becoming more physically active, she shared that she was feeling better about herself.

Intermediate phase (sessions 6 to 15): Throughout the work stage, Barb continued to talk about the work she was doing on the goals in her life outside of the group. The therapist encouraged Barb to notice her style of glossing over problems. Barb also received productive feedback from other group members about minimizing her feelings. Highlighting these repeated difficulties in the group interaction and linking them to a pattern in her outside relationships were essential in moving her work forward. Meanwhile, as Barb spoke about her unhappiness during her first marriage, she began to understand that maintaining the façade of a perfect life prevented her from turning to others for assistance. She began to see that by discounting her feelings, she prevented herself from experiencing her emotions or dealing with her feelings in more adaptive ways. This disconnection from self and others would appear in her group behavior. As it occurred in the group, members and leaders could address these issues with her in the moment.

The progression of the group through the conflict stage provided Barb with further opportunities to observe that conflict could be worked through effectively. When two group members had a conflictual interaction and were able to resolve it, Barb was able to learn in a concrete way how the expression of feelings can result in increased connection rather than isolation. And the successful resolution of a few instances of friction between herself and others in the group helped her to see that disagreements can have positive outcomes, such as helping her feel affirmed and improving the quality of her relationships. Outside of group, too, Barb began to share openly with her sisters, to communicate more with co-workers, and to set limits with clients when necessary.

Termination phase (sessions 16 to 20): By the last phase of treatment, Barb was aware of the enormous amount of energy she had expended in trying to conceal her problems; she was also sharing more with family and friends. As a result, she reported feeling closer to others. In fact, she and her boyfriend had become engaged. She continued to decrease her work hours. She had frank discussions with her daughters about their feelings toward their father. Having learned to recognize her emotions and take care of herself, she was better able to handle negative emotions as they arose. A continued goal for her to work on was giving more thought to conflict when it occurred rather than waiting for it to go away. She had stopped binge eating by the end of treatment and, at the eight-month follow-up, reported that she continued to be binge free.

Having a group member with the problem area of interpersonal deficits may be challenging at times for therapists. It is imperative that they ensure that this group member does not become a scapegoat. In addition, they will find it fruitful to monitor their own and other participants' potentially negative reactions to the member's style of relating. At the same time, the work of the ID member must not be allowed to repeatedly disrupt the work of others in the group. It is essential for the therapist to model how to give feedback in a gentle way that targets interpersonal behaviors, not the person. An attempt to treat interpersonal deficits in a short-term model may be difficult. It is helpful to emphasize that some members will only be able to begin work on these issues and will not necessarily resolve them by the group's end.

GROUP FACILITATION IN THE INTERMEDIATE PHASE

Many patients with depression and eating disorders share an interpersonal style of avoiding the expression of negative feelings due to fears of rejection. The group becomes an ideal setting where they can experiment with discussing these feelings and receiving feedback on their acceptability. These interactions contribute to acquiring skill in the successful resolution of conflict, which the therapist can promote both directly and by encouraging other members to provide input. Continual illumination and understanding of the group members' process is central to recovery.

In order to facilitate a relatively free discussion of material, the therapist should use general open-ended questions, especially in the early part of a session. More detailed inquiry can occur as the session progresses and members join in the discussion. For instance, "Say more about your relationship with your partner" could be followed by progressively more specific questioning.

MARKING THE END OF
THE INTERMEDIATE PHASE

Members, it is hoped, have been busy during this phase of treatment as they have worked toward their goals. Strong group cohesion facilitates work outside the session, leading to feelings of accomplishment and success. Overall, the IPT-G therapists endeavor to achieve a focus on each patient's current interpersonal problems as manifested in the group and in outside social life. Their primary goals are to challenge and encourage members to alter maladaptive interpersonal relationships—again, both within and outside the group. The group provides an optimal setting in which to explore and understand the ways in which members relate to one another and approach or avoid intimacy and confrontation (i.e., through interpersonal learning).

By the end of this phase, members are acutely aware that the group will soon be ending. This knowledge may bring up considerable anxiety. The therapist can formally bring this phase to an end by saying something like the following:

> Today's session marks the end of the intermediate phase of treatment. Part of what we need to do today is reflect on what has been achieved in terms of your goals and express any feelings regarding the ending of this stage. We still have time to work on your goals, so you can spend some time today talking about what is left to do. It is also important to comment on the changes that you see in each other and to discuss the feelings that accompany that aspect of your work together.

It is imperative that all group members participate in this discussion of feelings and outline what still needs to be accomplished before the group's end. In the process, the group's energy will be channeled in a productive way that can carry through the termination phase of treatment.

CHAPTER 6

The Termination Phase

The termination phase is an essential component of IPT treatment. On a basic level, it is a specified stage during which members are given a chance to consolidate progress, formally say good-bye, and discuss concerns about relapse and the possible need for future treatment. On a more poignant level, it is a time when members must learn to manage the emotions associated with ending relationships that they have found useful and meaningful. Hence it is a time when many complicated and conflicted feelings are brought up. The ways in which members grapple with this latter issue will determine how the basic tasks of the termination phase are approached by each of them. When this aspect of treatment is managed successfully, it can promote motivation and application that continue long after group ends.

The termination phase is considered to encompass the last five sessions. During this significant stage of treatment, therapists encourage the group to address several themes central to the termination process:

- recognizing that termination is a time of possible loss, an analogue of grieving;
- acknowledging negative reactions regarding not getting enough treatment or being abandoned;

- emphasizing the progress that each member has made, especially in terms of improved relationships and socialization outside of group;
- maintaining the stance of adopting personal responsibility for continued work on problem areas;
- discussing concerns about future need for treatment; and
- specifically saying good-bye to each other and to the therapist(s).

DISCUSSING
TERMINATION EXPLICITLY

The therapist must systematically raise the issue of reactions to impending termination in each of the last several sessions. Sometimes these themes emerge spontaneously in the group, in which case the therapist can reinforce an exploration of them at those times. Repetition of this task is generally required, as group members often avoid a direct discussion of the meaning of termination. Initially, some may not be aware of having feelings about termination. Introducing the idea that termination is an explicit stage will plant the seed that it is an important topic to discuss. The intensity of termination reactions will vary according to the length of time that the group has been meeting and the level of group cohesion achieved. However, even in less intense groups, termination will activate personal responses that need to be acknowledged and worked through. It is useful to bear in mind that therapists also react to impending termination. Indeed, this section has been designed in part as a guide to prevent therapists from postponing talk of termination. Therapists need to conceptualize termination as a formal part of the treatment package that carries with it many powerful therapeutic ingredients.

Before the group concludes, members need to be given many opportunities to reveal their feelings about termination and the ways they are managing it. In some cases, group members will begin a productive discussion of feelings once termination is mentioned. In others, one or two members may say something and the group will return to work-stage issues. It is useful to let the members work out how they would like to handle this aspect of treatment. If the group seems to be attending to the necessary tasks of this phase and continuing to work on themes related to termination of the group, the therapist can be less active. However, well before the last group, the therapist needs to make sure that the principal termination themes have been raised and that all members have participated in the discussion. This phase can be introduced in the following manner:

THERAPIST: The next five sessions mark the last phase of IPT. We'll be taking time to consolidate our work together and point out changes you have all seen in each other. We can reflect on what has been done and talk about what is left to do. This group has been important to all of you in different ways. It is important to talk about what it's like to have the end of the group in sight. Many of you may experience feelings of sadness, apprehension, and even anger as we prepare to wrap things up. It is important that each of you talk about these feelings. . . . What have people been thinking about or feeling in terms of the group ending?

A POTENTIAL TIME OF GRIEF

Reactions to the group's conclusion are often varied. As the group nears completion, and sometimes well before that, members may develop anxiety about saying good-bye to each other and going it alone. Since termination marks the end of a connection to other group members and the therapist, it has a theme of loss, an analogue of grief. It is important to state this possibility explicitly, as unacknowledged sad feelings may lead to fears of relapse and an increase in symptoms.

It is common for people with psychological difficulties to be particularly sensitive to perceived loss. Indeed, some members with issues of abandonment or feelings of isolation will have voiced fears about the group's ending early on, in the initial or intermediate phases of treatment. Even though the therapist reiterates the short-term nature of the group, and helps members to recognize progress in each session, many may fear that once they leave this supportive environment, their symptoms will return and/or they will not be able to retain the gains they have made. It is not uncommon to hear some members report a reemergence of symptoms similar to those that brought them into treatment. The therapist must recognize that working through each of these concerns is the task of the termination phase.

Equally important is noticing when termination-related issues and feelings are being broached in the group's discussion. For example, members may raise issues about death or loss without tying them to concerns about the group's end. The therapist should take this opportunity to guide members in a discussion of their feelings about the "death" or loss of the group, as in the following example:

> In the seventeenth session of the group, a member began discussing the upcoming move of one of her neighbors. She explained that she had just started to get to know these neighbors over the past few months, only recently finding out they were planning a move in the near future. She discussed her feelings of sadness and remorse that she hadn't extended herself more to them. Another group member joined the discussion by stating that he regretted not keeping in touch more with his brother who had moved with his family to another state. The therapist gently directed the members to reflect upon how those feelings might be related to the feelings they had about the upcoming ending of the group.

NEGATIVE FEELINGS
ABOUT TERMINATION

One aspect of termination that frequently concerns therapists is that talking about it may elicit negative feelings toward them. They may feel a strong inclination to add a few more sessions "just in case," to delay addressing termination themes, or to initiate talk about making further plans for treatment. It is important to remember that members will react to an imposed ending, even though they have known about it from the beginning.

The therapist should therefore move confidently toward the termination task, which must include both positive and negative dimensions of the group's ending. A hesitant or apologetic stance will interfere with constructive termination. Encouraging members to verbalize the negative dimensions allows for cognitive mastery of them so that they do not go underground and remain as a resentful residue of the therapeutic experience. Inevitably, members will also bring up positive dimensions of the termination experience, such as being able to identify unrealistic expectations and feeling some excitement at the prospect of moving on with their lives:

> With only two more sessions remaining in a group for members with major depression, a woman whose depression was related to the untimely death of her husband expressed her fear that she was getting depressed again. In an angry tone, she stated that she felt that she had received no benefit from the group and was going to leave feeling just as bad as when she had started. The therapist encouraged her to say some more, which she did. Two other members chimed in on the same theme. At that point another group member pointed out how hard all three had worked to make obvious changes while in the group. Another said she was actually looking forward to having her Wednesdays free again. The session ended on that note.
>
> The following session began with the initial woman saying that she had been thinking about what she had said last week. She realized that it was the same reaction she had when her husband had died. She felt that her hurt and anger couldn't be put into words because doing so would dishonor her husband's memory. During the week she had stood in front of her husband's picture and yelled that she was mad as hell that he died and she still loved him. All in the room were close to tears.

An important message to convey is that everyone must experience loss and address the associated feelings of not getting enough from their environment. Learning to work through these feelings is, in essence, a matter of learning to address the human condition.

PROGRESS REVIEW

Another important aspect of ending the group is encouraging members to talk about the progress they have made and the changes they have witnessed in each other, thus helping to consolidate the work that has been done. It is common for group members to easily identify improvement in others but not in themselves. Depression, for example, brings with it a predisposition to see the self in negative or critical terms. Members with eating disorders are quick to attribute change to the efforts of others or to circumstances, not to their own efforts. Crediting each member for changes that have been made is important because members may want to attribute these changes to the therapists. Indeed, such misplaced credit could erode the members' confidence in their continued success and improvement without treatment.

As members review their own and each other's progress, an increase in self-confidence usually occurs. The therapists need to emphasize how members have begun to successfully manage their relationships outside of group. From the start, members have received the message that the group is not a substitute for these outside relationships but, rather, was formed to assist members in learning how to deal with them. Members can be directed to recognize that these outside resources are now more available to them due to the effort they have invested in making better use of their social environment. The basic message is that it's important for patients to assume responsibility for monitoring their own lives, their relationships, and their involvement in social activities.

MAINTAINING
THERAPEUTIC GAINS

Each member should identify areas that need further attention, as some goals will not have been accomplished within the group's time frame. Future difficulties (including self-criticism, negative mood, and overeating) can be expected, so the therapist needs to cultivate a discussion of how to handle them. By discussing these issues openly, the members will receive the message that continued change and progress require efforts similar to the work they have already been doing. Predicting that setbacks will occur helps members to be realistic about change. It also underlines the fact that continuing benefits will involve accepting personal responsibility for application. This is an important theme that works against passivity and undue reliance on others, whether therapists or family and friends.

Guiding members in a discussion of contingencies for handling future problems will bolster feelings of competence. It is vital to assist members in thinking about warning signs and symptoms that suggest a need for future treatment. The therapist may recommend that they discuss these indicators with significant others as such indicators can help the members notice changes in much the same way as occurred in the group. In addition, specific action strategies should be rehearsed and perhaps written down.

Members with eating problems can be encouraged to view their symptoms as a vulnerability or an "Achilles' heel." This understanding may help to foster a realistic expectation about eating behavior. Specifically, it is important for members to realize that when they are having social or emotional difficulties, eating may be one of the first ways that they attempt to cope. Once they recognize the eating as a sign of distress and can put into practice alternative ways to cope, they will be less likely to turn a single episode of binge eating into a pattern of binge eating.

Members with major depression need to know that if they have experienced several episodes of depression, they are highly likely to have further episodes. Such members must therefore consider the types of triggers they have found and prepare themselves for addressing them. They must also be alert for early signs of depression so that they can seek treatment at an early point. Some will find it helpful to make an "emergency response" card that lists these recommendations.

BRINGING THE INITIAL
CONTRACT TO AN END

Termination is often a time of discomfort. Inevitably, some members will suggest that the group get together outside of the clinical setting and there will be a flurry of telephone number exchanges. The therapist may suggest that the group explore what they want to get out of the reunion. Such get-togethers seldom last long. The therapist needs to maintain a calm firmness about the ending of the group and the importance of talking about it. It is useful to emphasize that the group, as the members have known it, will no longer exist. They will need to say their good-byes and come to terms with this aspect of treatment.

It is also useful to introduce some structure to the final meetings, as was done in the beginning sessions. In the penultimate session, the members should be asked to think about what they would like to say to each of the other members by way of saying good-bye during the last session. For an eight-member group this process will often take up to an hour or more. The last session provides a formal opportunity to say good-bye and, equally important, to acknowledge the value of working with others in the group. This session is thus a rich source of empathic acknowledgment that is very enhancing to self-esteem. At the very end, it is best for the therapists to direct their remarks to the whole group, not to individual members. Following is a brief vignette taken from the final session of a group for members with binge eating disorder:

THERAPIST: Today we'd like to take time to give feedback to each other about changes made during the course of group. Why don't we start with Marilyn. You've done quite a bit of work and had a breakthrough with your husband.

MARILYN: I did make some good changes in my relationship with my husband, but I don't feel I've made as much progress as I should have or could have if I had taken better advantage of the group.

THERAPIST: Well, you took the time to make connections between your relationships and food. You stuck with it even though initially you weren't sure how it even applied to you.

MARILYN: I did. I let go of caretaking more, too. I realized I have to take care of myself and that no one will do that for me.

THERAPIST: What have others noticed with Marilyn?

TED: I've seen a shift in you. Even in group you changed, not apologizing as much but being more direct.

THERAPIST: How about you, Ted? What do you think about your own progress?

TED: I've gotten some tools. . . . I don't doubt myself as much, so I am more clear with other people now. My relationships at work are better, I think, because I work hard to be more aware of what I think and not to so easily just take on the opinions of others. I feel more confident and others respond to that.

THERAPIST: Other feedback for Ted . . . ?

Group members are encouraged to continue in this vein until all have commented on their own and each other's progress. The session ends with the therapist's comment:

THERAPIST: We were struck by the level of commitment and risk exhibited by everyone in the group. It has been this risk taking and commitment to change that have led to everyone making important changes. We encourage each of you to keep working on the goals that you have set. In many respects the real work begins today. It is a pleasure to have been a part of this process with you. We look forward to our individual meetings with each person.

FOLLOW-UP VISIT

Four to six months after termination, a follow-up visit with each individual member provides an opportunity to assess level of functioning. It also serves as an incentive for the patient to continue with the work begun in the group. If questionnaires were used at assessment, they can be used here as well. For those members who have not responded to treatment, or have truly relapsed, arrangements for additional treatment can be made at this time.

In summary, termination is a time of transition. It marks the end of one format for change and a movement toward the beginning of another: life after group, when members must "become their own therapist." Unless a crisis situation emerges, members should be encouraged to live with the results of their treatment and to avoid seeking further psychotherapy until after the follow-up visit. They should also be told that they can expect to continue to see progress with their goals after the group ends, provided that they continue to actively address the issues they have been dealing with throughout the group. This ongoing process of change is well reflected in the outcome literature.

PART FOUR
CLINICAL AND
TRAINING ISSUES

CHAPTER 7

Group Facilitation
in IPT-G

IPT-G TECHNIQUES

This section describes a number of basic group facilitation techniques that are available to the IPT-G therapist. The group therapist will need to decide when it is appropriate to use these techniques based on such factors as the stage of group, member readiness, and problem area(s). What makes IPT-G distinct is not the use of these standard group interventions but, rather, the strategies involved in addressing each of the four problem areas. Note that many of the examples involve bringing in group members to address the problematic issue in question.

Maintaining the Focus on Current Application:

Keeping a focus on current interpersonal relationships is the unifying theme throughout the intermediate sessions. The group therapist must constantly keep in mind each member's problem area and associated goals. Sessions do not pass without reference to these goals. The target goals form (see Table 3.3 in Chapter 3), which provides a concise summary of the goals, can be reviewed regularly before group sessions. As the depth of work increases, it is expected that members will encounter resistance to addressing the problematic issues that brought them into treatment. Therapists need to be as active as necessary to refocus the discussion. This is best done at an early point rather than letting off-focus discussion continue for too long. Vague, unfocused, or symptom-laden discussions are diverted as a way of refocusing members on specific and personal accounts of the problems being addressed. Tangential discussions also need to be interrupted or related to the central themes and goals of treatment. In this way, topics of personal emotional importance to the members will be emphasized whereas discussions of an abstract, technical, or intellectual nature will not be. Continuously reinforcing the connections among members and highlighting their relevance for all parties are important aspects of conducting IPT-G.

GROUP EXAMPLE

In session 6, several members with a similar history of childhood abuse began to challenge the group therapists about the limiting focus of the group. They were concerned that the group would not be able to help individual members manage some very painful early experiences and their associated emotions, which they felt were related to their current symptoms. Although the therapists permitted some discussion of their concerns, members were guided to consider how the patterns that began with the early trauma continue to reverberate and are perpetuated in present-day relationships. Making changes in the present does not mean trying to rewrite the past or block it out, but it does mean shifting the focus of the work to the present. There is clearly not enough time for all members to go into great detail about their past experiences. In an empathic manner, the point must be made that moving the working focus into the present will be most helpful to members striving to recuperate from their current symptoms. Indeed, by focusing on treatment goals and on improving their relationships, members can recover and feel more in control of their lives. Consider the following excerpt from session 6:

THERAPIST: It's been very helpful to understand how difficult a time it was for John to manage when his parents separated and he was more or less left on his own with distant relatives. And it's easy to see how his style of being resolutely independent, though lonely, came about. Does anyone see a connection to how this relates to his current relationship difficulties?

As noted in Chapter 5, to facilitate a relatively free discussion of material the therapist should use general open-ended questions, especially in the early part of a session. Then, as the session progresses and members join in the discussion, more detailed inquiry can occur. For instance, "Say more about your relationship with your partner" could be followed by progressively more specific questioning.

LINKING PROBLEM AREAS

Although there are four problem areas in IPT-G, each with a different set of goals and strategies, they all fall under the umbrella of interpersonal relationships. Group members will describe a variety of such issues as they work on their problems. Therapists can facilitate the working process by continuously linking one member's work with another if the members are not actively doing so. Each of the four IPT problem areas share some strategies with others. For example, the tasks of developing or reestablishing social relationships and exploring feelings associated with the problem context apply to all four. The problem areas of *grief* and *role transitions* both emphasize the importance of a realistic review of the status before and after the stressful event in order to achieve perspective on the changes required; *interpersonal disputes* and *interpersonal deficits* often involve similar types of difficulties in socialization.

All group members can benefit from reflecting on how another member's issue, from one of the other IPT problem areas, may relate to their own lives, even if it is not a primary concern at this time. In fact, many members will have a secondary problem area to address. For instance, someone may present to treatment with role transition as a primary problem area, but a role dispute may be a secondary concern or may arise during the course of understanding issues in the transition situation. The point is that usually there will be more than one member dealing with a particular problem area or target goal so that common work can be encouraged between them.

GROUP EXAMPLE

In session 12, Dan (problem area: role transition) began by letting the group know that he was not doing well. He went on to share that he had learned yesterday that one of his father's closest friends had committed suicide. Given his recent relocation, he was feeling guilty about not being able to be more available to his father during this time. As he discussed his feelings of guilt, sadness, and anger at his dad's friend, a woman in the group (problem area: abnormal grief) became quite upset with feelings of shock and anger. Her issues were directly connected to the situation of Dan's father, and she revealed many painful details concerning the sudden death of her mother two years ago. Another group member (problem area: interpersonal disputes) who had experienced passive suicidal ideation during the course of the group also found herself expressing feelings about her difficulties acknowledging alternatives to suicide when managing her own life issues. The therapist identified the group theme that emerged as "What do I do with all these feelings?" In talking together in the session, all members learned that part of the recovery process is realizing that you can tolerate emotions without resorting to maladaptive behavior.

HARNESSING MEMBER-TO-MEMBER RELATIONSHIPS

The group environment provides an opportunity for members to notice and comment on their reactions to each other. Such interactions may include confrontation and clarification, as well as support. This dimension of group psychotherapy also heightens the potency of IPT strategies that involve the member becoming aware of his or her own contribution to the development of unsatisfying encounters with others. Consider, for example, a member whose marital disputes derive in part from a "caretaking style" in which she gives priority to others' needs, only to boil over later from resentment and feelings of deprivation. She will typically experience similar difficulties in the group—initially not claiming time or attention for herself, but later finding herself feeling alienated, irritable, and ready to drop out of treatment. The therapist can actively promote the expression, examination, and management of such difficult feelings.

Many patients with depression and eating disorders share an interpersonal style of avoiding the expression of negative feelings due to fears of rejection. The group becomes an ideal setting where they can experiment with discussing these feelings and receive feedback on how well they have expressed themselves—a process that contributes to acquiring skill in the successful resolution of conflict. The therapist can promote this process both directly and by encouraging other members to provide input. Continual illumination and understanding of the group members' process is central to recovery.

It is helpful to begin exploration of intermember tensions with general open-ended questions, especially in the early part of a session. More detailed inquiry can occur as the session progresses and members join in the discussion. For instance, "Say more about your relationship with your partner" could be followed by progressively more specific questioning along the lines of "What exactly do you do when your partner makes a sarcastic remark?"

GROUP EXAMPLE

In session 10, Jan was able to directly address issues related to misunderstandings that occurred in the group between herself and two other members. Jan pointed out that she had distressing reactions to the response she had received during the previous session when she had shared some difficult feelings with Ann. Jan said that she experienced the feedback as rejection similar to what she has felt in the past.

Historically, when Jan had gotten her feelings hurt, she pulled away and disconnected herself. After she shared these feelings, several members began to support her opinions and feelings as valid. Rather than withdrawing or holding onto hurt feelings, she was active in trying to resolve them with other group members. By allowing herself to share her painful reactions, she was directly able to challenge the belief that she would be discounted or pushed away. She also gave others the opportunity to express their point of view and clarify what they had meant by their comments.

By checking things out, listening to feedback, and expressing reactions, members can use the group as a tool that they then apply to real-life issues that inevitably come up in interpersonal relationships. Before the next session, Jan had a significant transfer of learning based on her group experience. When she and her daughter got into an argument, she decided to stay and talk it out instead of leaving and getting into a stew about it later. Her daughter responded positively to the discussion, and they were able to go out together later with the air cleared.

CLARIFICATION

The short-term goal of this technique is to make members more aware of what they have actually communicated. Some examples follow.

1. Ask a group member to repeat or rephrase what has been said. This is particularly useful when a group member has said something in an unusual way or you want to highlight a connection that he seems to be making.

THERAPIST: John, could you say that again? It sounded like it had a lot of meaning for you.

Clarification is also helpful when a conflict arises among group members. By slowing members down, it allows them to explore the meaning of their feelings.

THERAPIST: What was it about Joe's statement that led you to feel rejected?

2. Call attention to contradictions in the presentation of material. For example, there may be a contradiction between the member's affective expression and her verbal discussion.

THERAPIST: Joan, I seem to be getting two messages: One is information about this awful situation you find yourself in, and the other is that you are smiling as you describe it. Have others noticed that?

3. Discrepancies can also be noted when material is discussed in a manner that contradicts earlier material.

THERAPIST: Joan, please help me to understand that you said _____ when previously you had said _____.

COMMUNICATION ANALYSIS

This technique is used to identify communication difficulties and to help members learn to communicate more effectively. After asking a member to recall in detail a recent interaction or argument she had with a significant other, the therapist can identify difficulties in communication and the underlying assumptions that the member makes about others' thoughts or feelings. The therapist can also ask other members for their reactions or connections to the speaker. Any repeated patterns in the member's in-group behavior can be punctuated. Alternatives to poor communication can be suggested after an exploration of associated issues.

GROUP EXAMPLE

In session 14, Joan began by sharing that she had had a difficult week, yet was unclear about what was going on for her. She mentioned an increase in her symptoms and said that an "I don't care" attitude permeated her affect. Joan had spoken to a former partner during the week and was encouraged to talk in detail about the interaction. It became clear that Joan was quite anxious about what her former partner might be feeling and thinking about her, and that she had put up a "front" in an effort to hide her disappointment at how their business had split up—a situation for which she blamed her partner. Other members were quick to note how Joan avoided the real issue and invited Joan to tell them what she really wanted to get out of the discussion. Those with similar styles joined in the discussion. Joan was encouraged to draw her own conclusions about the interaction *before* others joined the discussion.

ENCOURAGEMENT
OF AFFECT

Learning to become aware of internal feelings (i.e., clarification) is followed by learning to express, accept, and understand what they mean. A number of therapeutic techniques are available to this end. Two such techniques involve prompting the member (1) to acknowledge and accept painful affects and (2) to use her affective experience to bring about desired interpersonal changes.

The first of these techniques is facilitated by the group, which provides an arena in which to experience and express feelings. Many group patients are emotionally constricted in situations where strong emotions would normally be felt. They may be unassertive and not feel anger when their rights are violated. Or they may feel anger but lack the courage to express it in a direct manner. In such cases, it is important for the IPT-G therapist to help members acknowledge their feelings. One way to do this is to encourage other members to share experiences in which they have felt similarly: "Is anyone else connecting with what Mark is feeling?" If members deny being upset, even though it is clear that an upsetting interaction has just occurred, the therapist might say, "Although you said you were not upset, it appears that you have shut down since Mary said that to you. Have others noticed that Mary has shut down?"

The second technique—teaching how to use affect in interpersonal relationships—begins with identification of the affect being felt and the experience it is connected with. The next step is to activate the emotion within the group setting. The goal is to help group members act more constructively in interpersonal relationships. Depending on the circumstances, this may involve either expressing or suppressing affect. In other words, by learning to identify, understand, and acknowledge their feelings (whether or not they choose to verbalize them to others either in or outside of group), members can distinguish between real-life situations that are best managed by expressing affect and those that are best met by suppressing affect.

GROUP EXAMPLE

Sandy (problem area: role disputes) had spent some time in group discussing difficulties she encounters when interacting with her immediate family members. Meanwhile, others in the group noticed that Mike (problem area: role disputes) had become silent and withdrawn. Initially, he denied what other members saw as they commented on his nonverbal behaviors. But the group was persistent, and he eventually acknowledged that he was feeling hurt because his father had not acknowledged his son's first birthday. He spent some time clarifying and expressing his feelings of anger and rejection with regard to his own relationship with his father. The theme that the group adopted, with minimal direction from the therapist, became "When do you stop wanting something from a parent that you can never get?" Even though Mike became aware of and expressed many painful feelings regarding his relationship with his father, it was not his goal at this time to express these feelings to his father directly. Instead, members began to discuss how they could become more fulfilled and satisfied by working to make other choices in terms of who they turn to for support and companionship.

SUPPORTING POSITIVE
APPLICATION AND EVALUATION

In general, it is better to encourage members to examine feelings and expectations first, before moving on to try out new behaviors. Once new behaviors are attempted, the group can help individual members to evaluate the outcome and decide whether a different course of action is needed. Ongoing assessment of progress and highlighting change are necessary and valuable aspects of group work, in that they can help members to translate in-group discussions to outside application in their daily lives.

GROUP EXAMPLE

In session 10, the midpoint of the group, the therapist suggested that members take some time to share with each other about some of the changes they had made and the goals they wanted, and needed, to be working on over the remaining ten weeks. The therapist also suggested that members discuss how the changes they had made in their outside lives was affecting their symptoms. At that point, Wendy talked about how important it is for her to begin to share things more spontaneously in group. She described how, at times, she sits in group and waits and waits for the right time to speak, filtering what she wants to say and eventually feeling quite frustrated. She reported that she had become aware that she interacts the same way in most of her relationships. The therapist commented on this increased self-awareness and noted that there was still time left in the group to address these patterns in her life, but that she needed to begin making efforts to change. In session 11, Wendy pushed herself to risk being more open despite her reservations and managed her anxiety by checking in with the group about how she was coming across. Group members let Wendy know that she seemed more "real" and "honest" and that they liked her that way. Tim, who was also struggling with allowing himself to be more open, modeled his behavior on Wendy's example. By the following session, both Wendy and Tim were able to describe ways in which they pushed themselves to be more open with significant others and the positive effect it had on mood and self-esteem. Other members were supportive of their efforts.

SUMMARIZING

A review of important group themes that emerge during a session can have a supportive, clarifying, and unifying effect on group members. Sometimes a member will spontaneously provide a summary. At other times one of the therapists will comment on significant themes. In some group formats, the therapists will provide a written summary of the session.

GROUP EXAMPLE

At the end of session 15 in a twenty-session group, the therapist commented on several themes that members were addressing:

> THERAPIST: A significant issue that came up for members over the last several sessions is how difficult it is at times to not only know what your feelings are, but to be able to clearly express them in the context of important relationships. Historically, members have worked to keep feelings pushed away. What we have seen happen since the group began is that members are much more aware of their feelings and have been finding ways to express them. As you work to change and improve your relationships, you need to become more open about your feelings and more direct about what you want. Since for many this is a different way to be in relationship, it is bringing up a certain amount of fear and anxiety. As with other things, it takes practice. Part of the recovery process is to continue to find ways to be explicit and deliberate about your wants and needs.

MANAGING CHALLENGING
PATIENTS IN IPT-G

Certain patient behaviors may impede the group therapy process if not addressed promptly and thoughtfully. This section reviews some of these commonly encountered behaviors and offers methods of managing them in IPT-G. The therapist will need to monitor the norms that guide group participation and redirect members who demonstrate the behaviors described, keeping in mind that it is important not only to curb the problematic behavior but also to relate it to the interpersonal difficulties that the member is experiencing in outside relationships. By the same token, group members need to be encouraged to make a direct connection between behavior in group and overall interpersonal group goals. As a general principle, the first step is to tactfully address the problematic issue with the patient involved. This approach can be expanded to encourage group discussion about the situation, what impact it has on group function, and how it might be understood and modified.

THE PATIENT IS FREQUENTLY
QUIET OR PASSIVE

When a group member is consistently reticent or wordless in sessions, a problem is created. Evidence indicates that members who eventually drop out of group tended to participate less frequently in sessions than those who complete treatment (Oei and Kazmierczak, 1997). Members who do not participate are less likely to benefit from group treatment when compared to those who are more self-disclosing and moderately active (Tschuschke and Dies, 1997; Tschuschke, MacKenzie, Haaser, and Janke, 1996). Other members may feel judged by a reticent member. And, finally, it is easier for other members to project negative characteristics onto the quiet member since the latter is more difficult to "read."

When the therapist explores this issue with the group members involved, they may respond by saying something like "I learn by observing." In such cases, the therapist needs to stress that all members, if they are to recover, need to push themselves to take group time to talk about themselves and their goals. There are a number of ways to assist members in being more open. Some examples follow.

1. Facilitate discussion by all members by initially linking them to each other and encouraging active participation.

> THERAPIST: Several of you have mentioned the goal of wanting to be able to talk more instead of holding onto your feelings. What is it like to try to work on that in here?

Comment on the quiet member specifically:

> THERAPIST: Jessica, you look like you have been listening, but you haven't said much today. What has been going on for you?

2. If the behavior continues, encourage the member to strive to work on this behavior in group by tying it to one of her goals. This is also a good way to foster interpersonal learning.

> THERAPIST: I know when you met with us in your pregroup interview, one thing we discussed was a tendency to hold onto your feelings. Then later, you'd find yourself binge eating. One goal was learning how to express your feelings at the time. That might be a good thing to try and do here too, push yourself to talk in group about how you are feeling right now.

Or

> THERAPIST: Anne, I notice you don't say much in group unless we directly address you or you wait until the last minute of the session. What makes you hesitant to join in the discussion?

The member may respond that she is afraid that she sounds "stupid" when she talks, or fears that others may not like her. Exploring these responses within the group can lead to a fruitful discussion of feelings. And pointing out the difficulties that arise from this behavior in group can stimulate members to think about its impact on outside relationships with significant others.

Sometimes, other group members are the best resource for encouraging involvement.

> THERAPIST: I have seen a number of you talk to Christine today. I wonder if you have any more thoughts about how you can make it easier for her to get started talking more about the issues she wants to address here?

THE PATIENT MONOPOLIZES

In every group, someone inevitably rises to the task of "getting things going." In early sessions this group member is much appreciated by therapist and other group members alike. At least *someone* is willing to open up. This initial benefit, however, turns into a deficit when the monopolizer begins to talk incessantly and others become irritated, often unsure of how to respond. It is clear that a monopolizing style, if not redirected, becomes a drawback to the goals of a short-term IPT group.

The member who is monopolizing needs to learn how to observe the effect of her behavior in terms of its interpersonal consequences and, then, how to alter it. At the same time, other members need to learn how to "take" group time for themselves as well as share time among each other. The group therapist can facilitate a balance by allowing the members and monopolizer to "hone" each other. The initial interventions send the message that all are expected to share and to monitor their own level of participation. Below are some examples of how to work with the monopolizer.

1. Stop the monopolizer and ask others to comment on how they are connecting to what the person is saying:

THERAPIST: You have said a lot, Theresa, and I'd like to stop you and bring some others in and see how they may be relating to the issues you are raising today.

2. Make a connection between what the monopolizer is saying and another group member's work:

THERAPIST: I think Carl was also talking about that issue in the last session. Carl, are you identifying with what Beverly is saying?

3. If the monopolizer does not respond to your more subtle interventions, and the behavior continues, comment more directly on the process itself. One approach is to ask the group member to observe her own behavior in group and to try to summarize what she wants to convey:

THERAPIST: Suzanne, you are saying a lot and I'm getting kind of overwhelmed with all the particulars. I wonder if you could try summarizing, in one or two sentences, what you most want us to know about you or your feelings right now.

4. Comment on the behavior itself, and foster interpersonal learning:

THERAPIST: Marcie, I notice you are often the first to respond in here and it is good that you are ready to work, but I wonder if you are aware of how others are connecting in to what you are saying or how they are reacting to you. Would you like to take some time to ask for others' feedback about how you are coming across?

The main objective here is to stop the person from setting herself up for rejection by other group members—specifically, by helping her to modify her interpersonal behavior. Equally important is the fact that, when other members are encouraged to give feedback, it should focus on the behavior and how they are affected by it. For example, instead of saying "Liz, you talk too much," encourage feedback such as "Liz, when you talk without stopping I feel shut out, like you don't want to let me in or to get close." By creating a trusting atmosphere, the therapist allows the monopolizer to reflect on what "all the talking" is about for her. Tying this behavior to difficulties in outside relationships or interpersonal group goals can lead to increased insight and, hopefully, to a change.

THE PATIENT IS OBSESSING OVER SYMPTOMS

One version of monopolizer is the patient who talks at length about his symptomatic status and how it is affecting his life. Initially the group may respond to this situation with understanding and compassion, but if it continues it can hamper the group and eventually lead to a hostile response from group members. The therapist needs to be increasingly firm at redirecting the topic to interpersonal issues.

Make a clear statement about how the effect of focusing solely on symptoms detracts from the important work on established interpersonal goals:

> THERAPIST: It sounds like you are continuing to have a difficult time, Henry. Our job here in the group, for everybody, is to look at ways of improving the quality of your lives, especially in regard to your relationships. As you work to shift your focus onto the interpersonal goals that we worked on together, the symptoms of depression that you are so concerned about will begin to fade. I'm afraid that your continued focus on the symptoms will actually make them worse, while it takes up all the energy and effort that's needed to work on making these important interpersonal changes.

The Patient Engages
in Storytelling

The storytelling client discusses outside people or circumstances at great length and with much detail. The result is that others learn less about the group member than about the member's acquaintances. Storytelling can seem a lot like monopolizing when it is used repetitively as a way to communicate. In early group sessions, getting some detail about significant others is important as a way to obtain background information about group members. However, after this background is briefly described, it is valuable to refocus members so that they begin sharing their inner feelings about or responses to their significant others rather than continuing to dwell on the details of the significant others per se.

If the storyteller in the group does not respond to initial efforts to refocus, the therapist should consider using the following techniques.

1. Educate about group process:

THERAPIST: It is more fruitful if you try to focus on personal feelings or reactions toward others as you work on your problem areas than if you try to explain a lot of the details about others who are not in the group.

2. Comment on the interpersonal consequences of the behavior:

THERAPIST: When you talk about your feelings or your reactions to significant others, I feel I get to know you better. When you spend a lot of time filling in details of a circumstance, I feel more distant from you.

3. Encourage others in the group to comment on their sense of connection to the storyteller:

THERAPIST: What was it like for others to hear Samantha talk about herself and not spend so much time on the details of the situation?

Of course, the therapist needs to be careful not to interrupt someone abruptly in a caustic fashion. By gently encouraging members early on to talk about feelings and reactions rather than lengthy details, the therapist sends the message that this is what makes for good group discussion.

THE PATIENT QUESTIONS OTHERS

Questioning in the group can become a way to engage others while keeping them at arm length. Members who relate to others in this way are most likely hoping to increase their connection to others. When used often, however, questioning has the effect of making people feel uncomfortable or on the "hot seat." The therapist will find it valuable to help the questioner refocus his attention on what he means to accomplish and find other ways to obtain what he wants from his relationships.

Sometimes a simple suggestion can work:

THERAPIST: Ask yourself how you are responding to Austin or what he is saying, and make a statement about that, instead of hitting him with a lot of questions. What would you like to say to him right now?

Encourage examination of interpersonal consequences:

THERAPIST: Robby, I can see you are interested in finding out more about Davis by asking so many questions, but I wonder how it feels to Davis to be put on the spot like this?

By encouraging an exploration of the meaning behind the questions, the therapist can help the questioner learn about his style of engaging others and how he comes across. And by teaching members to rephrase their questions as statements, the therapist can prompt both self-awareness and direct communication.

THE PATIENT IS HOSTILE

It is hoped that pretherapy screening will have screened out patients who are consistently and actively hostile and controlling; patients with severe personality disorders are usually not appropriate candidates in an IPT-G setting. Such screening does not, however, exclude patients who become hostile when triggered in a particular session or those who have more subtle ways of expressing hostility.

When a major angry disagreement occurs, the therapist's first step is to calm members down, by means of direct and firm statements if required. The therapist can then facilitate an exploration of the conflict from all group members, starting with clarification of feelings from those most immediately involved. This approach provides a fine opportunity in which to identify and begin to modify the management of interpersonal conflict. It would be counterproductive for the therapist to evade this responsibility and give the message that tensions cannot be addressed. The incident should almost always be brought up at the next session in order to determine the further reactions of members after they have had a chance to reflect on it. Discussions of in-group hostility can progress to an exploration of how hostility is exhibited or managed in outside relationships.

Following are several techniques for dealing with intragroup hostility.

1. Contain the escalation of the anger if this appears imminent:

THERAPIST: Elizabeth and Michael, I know the two of you have some important issues to sort out. But that can't be done if you're both bouncing off the wall with your anger. Now I'm asking you both to sit down and give yourself a few moments to get things under control. Then we can all look at what's been happening and how the issues can be addressed in a more constructive way. Does anyone have some initial ideas about this?

2. Process the issues raised, and recruit the active involvement of other members:

> THERAPIST: Now, we know that there has been some tension between Elizabeth and Michael for a while. And that seems to be based on each of them having assumptions about what the other is thinking of them. It would be helpful if the rest of the group could speak to this and give them something to think about. I'm asking them to listen to your comments and then to respond to what the group has said. This is actually a good chance for everyone to think about how they handle or don't handle anger in themselves or others.

3. When hostility manifests itself as sarcastic remarks, facial expressions, or mumbled jokes the behavior can be pointed out and its interpersonal consequences explored. For example:

> When Marie spoke, Jan often began acting bored and joking quietly with the member sitting nearby. When the therapist commented on this behavior, Jan replied that she was fine and was "sorry" for interrupting. As the group continued, the therapist noticed the same behavior and encouraged Jan to talk about what was going on with her when Marie spoke. Jan said that Marie reminded her of her passive sister who was always letting others step on her. Marie was helped to respond to Jan's forceful response by forbidding Jan to interrupt while Marie was talking. Through this exchange, both Jan and Marie gained insight into the ways they come across to others. Jan was also encouraged to separate her feelings about her sister from those she had for Marie.

Other modes of expressing hostility may include missing sessions, arriving late, or being silent. Ways to manage these behaviors, and more challenging interpersonal behaviors, are discussed elsewhere in the chapter.

THE PATIENT MISSES
SESSIONS OR ARRIVES LATE

Consistency of attendance is an important component in group therapy. Valuable time is lost when members who have missed a session or arrive late have to be brought up to date. Individual patients also tend to lose their momentum of working on goals when group sessions are missed. The norm of attendance should be discussed and agreed upon in the pregroup meeting with the stipulation that if a predetermined number of sessions are missed, the patient will need to discontinue participation. It is helpful to require that members who miss a session come in early to view the previous week's videotape of the group (if available). Group summaries (see Chapter 8) can also be helpful to those who miss sessions. Arriving late to sessions must be discussed and not tolerated, as such behavior creates a counterproductive norm in the group. To facilitate building productive group norms, the therapist should emphasize the importance of attending all sessions. In addition, members should be asked to call ahead if they will be late or unable to attend:

THERAPIST: We expect that you will attend each session and arrive on time so we can respect everyone's commitment to working on his or her interpersonal goals. Please call if you will be late.

Once group has begun, some members may experience impediments to group attendance such as childcare difficulties, late work meetings, and so on. The members should be encouraged to find a way to resolve these matters so that they can continue their participation in the group.

In other instances, previously prompt patients may begin to miss group sessions or arrive late. In such cases, it is likely that the behavior has meaning related to the group therapy context. For example, some patients may feel that they are not getting the help they need in the group and indirectly express it by arriving late. The therapist may approach the issue in this way:

> THERAPIST: Terri, what do you make of your lateness to group today?

Or,

> THERAPIST: What do you imagine its effect is on the group?

A discussion of the meaning of the lateness or missed sessions should ensue, with the therapist facilitating an exploration of its interpersonal context. Identifying the connections among group behavior, group goals, and difficulties experienced in outside relationships is the foundation of IPT-G:

> A member with the problem area of role transitions began to arrive late, saying he didn't think it mattered since he didn't talk much anyway. As the behavior was explored, he revealed that as he was trying to make new friends, he often believed they found him boring. He avoided these feelings by acting as if others did not matter to him either, leaving him feeling pretty isolated. One of his initial goals was to become more involved in his community, and he realized how these feelings were getting in the way. Other group members responded to his feelings of "not fitting in" by sharing their own experiences. He left the session feeling more supported and re-energized to work on this goal.

Members like the one described here can be encouraged to choose more direct methods of communicating their feelings and to develop more effective behaviors to get what they need in relationships.

If several members are arriving late, the reason is most likely related to dissatisfactions or tensions within the group. The therapist needs to bring this issue into the group for a full discussion:

THERAPIST: Over the last two sessions and again today, several members have arrived late, something that really has not happened before in the group. We need to discuss this. Does anyone have some ideas about this?

THE PATIENT IS SUICIDAL

Those with an acute, active suicidal threat should have been screened out from group participation and offered other treatment options. Once the group begins, however, a group member may express suicidal thoughts or feelings and these must be taken seriously. Other group members can be quite fearful of this type of admission, depending on its severity, and will want to know that the therapist is prepared to handle the situation in a safe manner.

In many instances a productive discussion of feelings can be encouraged in the group, leading to safe resolution of the suicidal feelings. Such an outcome is possible when the suicidal feelings and thoughts are relatively passive and judged to be less severe in terms of suicide risk factors. Of course, this is always a judgment call by the group therapist. The way to deal with this issue in an IPT-G setting is to assist the group member in exploring what is behind the suicidal feelings, especially how they relate to the interpersonal context. The member can also be encouraged to think of suicide as an attempt at problem solving and led to explore other methods to get what he or she needs. Meanwhile, other members who have had thoughts of suicide at some point in their lives may be willing to share their experiences, thus providing the supportive atmosphere needed to allow the issue to be clarified, managed, and resolved in the session.

In other, more severe or crisis cases, it may become clear to the therapist that the patient is not able to do any productive work in the group at the present time. When this situation occurs, the therapist can suggest, during the group session, that the patient meet with the therapist after the session. This lets other group members know that the patient will receive the care he or she needs. Later, if the patient is able to return to the group, it is important to discuss the incident and process it as described above.

Getting the member to agree to safety is imperative, even in "less severe" cases. The member can be told to keep the therapist informed about any increase in thoughts or feelings of suicide. This can be done by way of phone calls between group sessions and by touching base after the group session to further evaluate the extent of suicidal thoughts, feelings, or intent. If upon exploration of the suicidal feelings and thoughts the patient appears to require further evaluation, concomitant individual treatment, or hospitalization, the intervention in question should be arranged by the group therapist.

Other challenging member behaviors not described in this chapter may arise during the course of IPT-G. In such cases, the best course of action within an IPT framework is to explore the meaning of the problematic behavior in terms of its interpersonal context and relate it to the identified problem area.

CHAPTER 8

Techniques for Intensifying the Interpersonal Focus in IPT-G

All of the time-limited psychotherapy models emphasize the importance of therapist activity in promoting a consistent focus on targeted areas. In addition to this general therapeutic principle, a number of specific techniques have been developed for augmenting the focusing task. Some of the more commonly used ones are discussed in this chapter.

INTRODUCTION OF INFORMATION FROM THE INTERPERSONAL INVENTORY

During the early sessions of the group, members are encouraged to discuss the nature of the issues raised during the pregroup meeting and interpersonal inventory. In addition, to facilitate self-disclosure and establish connections among group members (vital for the development of cohesion), the therapist may find it very helpful to make reference to the pregroup material even when the patient has not introduced it. Given that IPT-G is a time-limited treatment, the therapist must be active in the first few sessions to assist the group members in forging important therapeutic norms. (In less structured long-term groups, therapists usually wait for this important material to emerge.) On the other hand, the decision to introduce pregroup material raises issues of confidentiality. Therefore, it is necessary to discuss such an eventuality during the assessment and pregroup meetings. Reference should be made to the desirability of having the patients thoroughly discuss the assessment findings as they get comfortable in the group, but also to the possibility of allowing the therapist the option to refer to this information, if relevant, to what may be happening in the group. In this way, the fact that the assessment is "open material" becomes clear to all concerned. Of course, the introduction of such material needs to be done with clinical skill. Obviously, issues that concern early childhood trauma or sexual orientation are the exceptions. In these cases, the therapist should negotiate a timetable with the patient as to when it might be effective to share this information (if at all). The therapist may do this by saying "Jill, when Sara was talking about the difficulties she is having with her husband, I was aware that you shared some similar experiences with me in the our pregroup meeting. What kind of feelings or reactions were you having as Sara was sharing just now?" Often this information is linked to a theme in the group process that will help the patient forge deeper connections with other members with similar issues or experiences. The important thing is that the expectations are clearly laid out during the individual assessment sessions.

GROUP SUMMARIES

The use of group summaries to assist in maintaining a focus for group work has a long history (Yalom, 1995). In addition to maintaining an important interpersonal focus, summaries encourage members to think about how the group is being used and how each member relates to the group events. They also provide ongoing education about understanding the group process. This idea of demystifying the process of psychotherapy is a common thread through much of the time-limited literature. Theoretically, such activities should increase the capacity of the members to use the group environment to its maximum therapeutic potential.

Summaries are best prepared according to a standard format. Some therapists, for example, provide a sequential history of the session, highlighting particularly important incidents. Others prefer to summarize major themes in the session and to pay less attention to specific episodes. Most use some combination of these two methods and may add clarifying or interpretive commentary. Too much generalization loses individual impact, and too much detail loses larger implications. In their commentary some therapists rely mainly on describing content, leaving consideration of the meaning to the members. Others emphasize process implications with a strong interpretive flavor.

The most significant decision is whether or not to specifically discuss each member's role in the session. One summary model, for example, describes the major thematic episodes in the session and relates how the members participate in relation to these. This approach is the most integrative in terms of relating group phenomena to the individual member's role in such phenomena, although it means that some comment regarding each member must be included for each issue. Another feature of this model is that it emphasizes the interpretive function of the therapist and thus can become quite complex. It also raises possible questions of confidentiality if others such as parents or spouses have access to the summaries. In any case, it is wise to use only first names or initials.

Summaries can serve a useful therapeutic function, but they need to be used with clinical wisdom. First, they may include information or perspectives that are upsetting to a member. If an event is described that includes two or three members, it is wise to routinely provide an opportunity for them to react to the description, as doing so will often deepen their understanding of it. Second, in cases where patients have totally missed important group events, either because they were anxious over the topic or process or because they entered a partially dissociated state, reading group summaries can provide them with important information or give them a perspective on the material they missed. Third, in larger groups a lot may happen in a short time, and summaries allow a more thoughtful review of events. Finally, summaries can play a quasi-interpretive role by raising possible meanings of events being described. In this way they can provide an opportunity for the therapist to increase the focus on sensitive issues such as anger or tension in the group and to suggest that the matter needs further discussion in the next session.

In the NIMH comparative treatment trial for binge eating disorder (Wilfley, 1999), group summaries were used in IPT-G as a way to maintain an intensive interpersonal focus on each member's work in the group. Although there are no empirical data from the NIMH trial indicating that the detailed summaries were additive, clinical impressions and commentary from patients suggest that they were invaluable. In practical terms, it is unlikely that time will be made available for lengthy summaries outside of academic research settings. However, a one- to two-page summary focused on general group themes or events would be realistic and can be generated in a standard post-session review. The following example of a group summary (for session 3, in which Rob and Jenny are the co-therapists) was taken from the NIMH comparative treatment trial for binge eating disorder. As with other vignettes in this manual, great care has been taken to conceal the identities of the participants.

Group Summary Example

This was an extremely valuable session which underscored the importance of clear communication, direct feedback, and making connections with others. Members shared that they had clearly been impacted by the notes, and the input given to Rob and Jenny was very helpful. Among the important themes that came up during this session, members spoke about the dilemma that arises around the strong desire to be cared for and respected by significant others and the difficulty of experiencing and managing the conflicting feelings in those relationships. In addition, members were very helpful throughout the group in sharing how the issues brought up by others impacted their own lives. In short, important work was done by all.

The session began with eight members present. Rob explained that Robert had called to say he couldn't come to group because he was obliged to remain at work due to a major staff reorganization. Rob then began the group by encouraging members to share about the important people and relationships, both present and absent, in their lives.

Jeanne began by sharing with the group that she had helped to put her father into an institution this week. As you may recall from the first session, Jeanne's father is mentally ill and has struggled with this condition for years. Not only has Jeanne had to tolerate the lack of stability, she has had to manage the feelings of shame she has about her father's illness. Given this, it was very important that Jeanne had begun to come to terms with her multitude of conflicting feelings about her father. By allowing herself to talk through her feelings with her husband instead of dismissing them, Jeanne was able to tolerate the emotional upheaval and shame that usually occur around the painful memories or circumstances associated with her father's mental illness. As a result of using this different strategy, Jeanne shared with the group that she did not binge eat. This was very important work for you, Jeanne. In addition, you shared with the group during the last session that you had spoken with your husband about his controlling style (which is one of your goals). It would be important to know how that is going and whether your openness with him about your feelings has been able to continue.

This good work really struck a chord with the rest of the group. While Jeanne spoke, Rose reached out to her, offering that she, too, had very conflicting feelings for her own mother who had been alcoholic. When Rose had finished sharing her feelings and reactions with Jeanne, Rob wondered if Helen was able to connect, given that one of her goals is to work on the conflicts she has with her mother.

With that, Helen began to share with the group that she had conflicting feelings about her mother with whom she currently lives. Whereas her mother had historically been the person to whom she felt the closest, she was also the one that Helen had the most conflict with and "hated" the most. Specifically, Helen shared that her mother's critical comments and inconsistency had caused Helen to never know what would keep her happy. In response, Helen tried to adapt herself in an attempt to keep her mother happy and to respond to her mother's moods. Helen provided the group with an example of how her mother gives her mixed messages. On the one hand, it would appear that Helen's mother wants her to be happy and healthy, yet will make comments to her regarding her weight and her involvement in the group.

It is not unusual for individuals who struggle with binge eating to have come from a background where messages were not consistent and were critical. As children, the way to manage this kind of environment is to try and make things better through working hard, being nice, and keeping your feelings to yourself. Unfortunately, the turmoil that occurs within needs to be managed in some way. For many, eating becomes one way to manage the inconsistency and the stress. As a result, these patterns of people pleasing and keeping feelings to yourself continue into adulthood and create problems in all areas of life. For Helen and for others in the group, these situations often led to binge eating.

It is great that Helen is beginning to talk about these issues. As she mentioned in the last session, being in the group and sharing was one of the most difficult things that she had ever done. In this regard, her work in this session was impressive. One explanation of her reactions from the last session may be due to the fact that Helen is allowing herself to have strong feelings (which is very different for her). As a result, the experiences from the last session would be overwhelming. It will be important, Helen, for you to continue to talk about these issues. It will also be important to begin (with the group's help) to find ways for you to communicate with your mother about the things that trouble you. She may not know the degree to which her comments cause you distress. Because it might be anxiety provoking to think about doing this, it will be important to talk about it in the group.

At this point, Rob invited Nancy to share reactions that she might be having as Helen spoke. Nancy indicated that she strongly related to

Helen. Similar to Helen's mother, Nancy's father has typically made critical comments at times when Nancy has been motivated to make changes, such as asking "Are you sure they can help you?" Nancy shared that this week her mother had contributed to her stress in a similar way. Nancy was eating dinner after a day of work. As her father began enumerating the problems with the house remodeling that had happened that day, Nancy noticed that she began to eat "more and more and faster and faster." At that moment, Nancy realized that the stress of having work done on her house and having her father give her the details was leading to her overeating. Nancy went on to share that this insight lead to a few days of reduced binge eating.

Nancy, you did good work by noticing that the increased stress contributed to your problems with binge eating. Becoming aware of the times in which you are "stress eating" is an important part in the recovery from binge eating. By being aware of these critical moments, you can make choices to manage your stress differently rather than turning to food. Although the changes in your binge eating did not last as long as you wanted, they were changes nonetheless. The connection that you made was significant. Continue to push yourself to be aware of these situations both at home and at work. The more you can do this, you will begin to notice more lasting changes in your binge eating. Similar to Helen, it will be important to use the group to begin thinking and practicing other ways to manage these situations. By doing this, you will be actively working on taking better care of yourself.

When Nancy had finished, Susan indicated that she too had made a connection with Jeanne. Specifically, Susan shared that she felt connected with Jeanne in that she seemed to understand the struggle she (Susan) was having with her daughter's mental illness. Susan went on to share her struggle of feeling manipulated by her daughter as she was moving (little by little) back into her home. While clearly compassionate about her daughter's problems, Susan expressed her frustration with her and her disappointment in herself for not setting clearer limits by allowing her daughter to manipulate her. Susan shared that her daughter has been argumentative with her about the apartment that she helped her find.

As she was sharing, Rob asked Susan how the group could help her. Susan responded that the opportunity to talk about her daughter's situation was very important. Susan shared again how hard she works to keep her daughter's mental illness a secret from her co-workers. Other than a group for parents and family of the mentally ill, there are very few places where Susan can be open about this. Although it is extremely important that Susan has the group to share her concerns with, it might be helpful for Susan to begin thinking about how she might begin letting others know about this difficult situation (which is one of her goals). By keeping it to herself, she has to struggle with it alone. Although Susan's concerns about her daughter being stigmatized by others may be justified, there may be a great deal of care and support waiting for her as well. This will be important to talk about.

Earlier in the group, Paula commented on how important it was for her to let others know her needs. Paula shared with the group that she had guests from Florida this week, and that she was really enjoying their visit. As Paula continues to share her needs with others, she may be less likely to feel burdened by them. This is important work, Paula. In addition, Rob and Jenny were aware that they gave you some feedback in the notes about how you come across. Specifically, they mentioned that you carry yourself with confidence, and, consequently, others may not know that you feel "needy" in any way. It would be important to hear what you thought about that, and whether that holds true for you.

Later in the group, as Susan spoke about her daughter, Paula found herself asking questions of Susan and wondering with Susan whether her daughter's return home was in reality a good thing for her. The concern expressed by Paula for Susan, although thoughtful, seemed to be fairly emotion-filled. When Rob checked in with Paula, it became clear that she was having a strong emotional reaction out of her own disappointment that her son had *not* chosen to live with her. Indeed, it was clear that Paula had connected with Susan about the desire of having the best for their children and the problems this gave rise to. Paula spoke painfully in describing her efforts to make everything perfect for her son. For example, Paula had worked so hard to plan every moment of their vacations that they caused her enormous stress and disappointment (she also had several binge eating episodes as a result). Paula conveyed an earnest desire to be respected and not manipulated by her son. As Paula was sharing, Susan wondered if Paula, similar to her, was attending to her son's needs with the exclusion of her own. As Rob suggested to Paula, one of her goals was to work toward expressing her feelings to her son and seeing where the chips may fall. Indeed, it will be important to talk with Paula about ways she feels she can get her needs met in the context of her relationship with her son.

The exchange between Paula and Susan was significant. Initially, Paula's questions and suggestion to Susan that her daughter's coming to live with her was a good thing seemed to create some distress for Susan. However, as Rob pointed out, Paula's expressions of concern were more related to her own distress about her son. Susan seemed to understand this, and it appeared to clarify the conflict. In many ways, this is what Rob attempted to highlight in the previous session. Paula's questions were not only a way for her to express concern for Susan, but a way for her to work through her own feelings with her son. Fortunately, Paula was able to get in touch with her feelings of sadness and her frustration with her son. As Paula was able to shift the focus onto the issue with her son, Susan did not end up taking Paula's questions as a criticism of her parenting.

These types of interactions occur constantly, and unfortunately they can at times lead to misunderstandings and conflict. Given this, it is important to work at trying to understand the feelings and reactions you are having as you listen to others in the group. Sharing your reactions and feelings promotes connection with others and a deepening of understanding between others.

Throughout the group, Tammy appeared to have been very connected with others. When Susan and Paula were sharing about their respective concern and love for their children, Tammy began to experience some very strong emotions. When Jenny checked in with her about this, Tammy shared that Paula's and Susan's concern had made her aware of how sad she felt inside. When Rob followed up with this, it became clear that Tammy had been touched by the care that Paula and Susan had expressed. Tammy shared that, in many ways, it would have been so good to have known that her father had cared for her in a similar way. Tammy went on to express that as a result of her reaction, she became very aware that there are still many conflicting feelings that need to be examined in relation to her father. Although this was very important, what seemed key was Tammy's ability to stay with her feelings of sadness and not try to push them away. This was important work in that it is proof that Tammy can express her feelings without being overcome by them. Tammy seemed surprised and pleased to feel as if "the stopper [of the emotions] came out." Tammy, it will be important to follow up with this.

As the session came to a close, Rob and Jenny checked in with group members who seemed to be feeling in a better place. This week members did very hard work revolving around the important people in their lives and caring for themselves in the context of their relationships. As Rob and Jenny mentioned, it will be equally important to hear about the lack of relationships or connections group members are feeling as well. Your feedback on the notes was extremely helpful. We want to make a special note that some group members had expressed that the way the notes were written caused them distress. Specifically, there seemed to be concern that the notes would become a way to confront or punish. We would like to stress that this is not the case. Clearly, the notes from the previous session (most notably the feedback to Rose) should have been stated differently and could have been given within the context of the group. It is hoped that this will be the rare exception and not the rule. With this in mind, it will continue to be important for members to let us know (as Samantha did) when things are said that create distress. In no way are the notes intended to be mean spirited. They are, and continue to be, a forum to encourage and support your continued work on your goals as you strive to recover from your binge eating.

Have a good week. We hope that the reorganization of staff went smoothly for Robert this last week. We look forward to seeing you next week.

The idea of reinforcing a thoughtful consideration of each session can also be addressed in less complex ways. For example, as discussed in Chapter 4, a wrap-up discussion is encouraged at the end of each session. This discussion provides a debriefing opportunity for both member and therapist input. It has the added advantage of picking up potentially distressing reactions that members may not have verbalized during the session itself. Similarly, a check-in at the beginning of each session could include a focus on further reactions that occurred in the interim between the last session and the current one. The therapist might have an informal agenda of core issues or themes to insert into this discussion. All of these techniques are in the service of encouraging continuity and maintaining a strong interpersonal focus.

SELF-HELP MANUALS

Another useful technique for intensifying the interpersonal focus of an IPT-G group involves the use of self-help manuals in conjunction with group treatment. With this model, all group members would be given manuals and instructed to read them over the course of treatment. There has been a growing awareness of the value of informing patients not only about the indications for the type of treatment being recommended but also about the nature of the treatment itself. In the case of IPT-G, this approach involves several areas of emphasis—the most important of which is a full review of the symptoms of the disorder being treated (e.g., major depression, bulimia nervosa, or binge eating). This review can be handled by means of a handout sheet listing the formal DSM-IV criteria for the syndrome under discussion.

Another useful technique involves discussion of the methods used in the treatment, including the sorts of strategies employed and how patients can best benefit from them in a collaborative process with their therapist. In terms of IPT, these goals are addressed in a self-help manual titled "Mastering Depression: A Patient's Guide to

Interpersonal Psychotherapy" (Weissman, 1995a). The first chapter of this slim paperback book provides an overview of the depressive syndrome in straightforward lay language. It also lists common questions about depression, including the possibility of self-harm. Chapter 2 gives a similar overview of how psychotherapy works—and, in particular, how IPT sessions will be conducted. Common concerns such as the role of the therapist and worries about what to talk about are addressed. The remainder of the book describes in some detail the sequence of events involved in the therapy. Major areas to be assessed, and the nature of the treatment contract, are reviewed. Then all of the four problem areas are described, along with the principal methods used to explore them. A companion publication, "Patient Assessment Forms Workbook for Interpersonal Psychotherapy Program for Depression" (Weissman, 1995b), provides a series of questionnaires related to IPT.

Although the use of self-help manuals in IPT-G has not been tested, it would appear to be a reasonable alternative strategy for maintaining the important interpersonal focus in IPT-G.

CHAPTER 9

Therapist Training
and Clinical Applications

THERAPIST TRAINING

Competence as an IPT-G therapist requires (1) a working knowledge of IPT theory and practice, (2) a working knowledge of group psychotherapy theory and practice, and (3) specific training in the concepts, strategies, and techniques of IPT-G.

TRAINING IN INTERPERSONAL PSYCHOTHERAPY

To receive training in individual IPT, the reader is referred to the *Comprehensive Guide to Interpersonal Psychotherapy* (Weissman et al., 2000). Although no formal certification process has been established, guidelines for training usually consist of a formal course or training workshop and detailed supervision from an experienced IPT clinician of at least two successfully treated cases. The IPT manual is well developed and describes the treatment process and its rationale in a manner that should be clear to any clinician. It should be noted that IPT was developed to serve as a semistructured guideline for clinicians who already possess a reasonable degree of clinical training and experience (Weissman et al., 2000). Clinicians planning to receive training in IPT-

G are advised to thoroughly familiarize themselves with the theory, concepts, strategies, and techniques of IPT, which are outlined in the new comprehensive text (Weissman et al., 2000), and to receive some training in individual IPT. (It is expected that the majority of those interested in IPT-G will already have been trained in IPT.)

Training in Group Therapy

It appears that graduates of professional training programs are generally expected to be able to conduct therapy groups. Yet, in actuality, training in group therapy is often nonexistent or extremely meager. Where it does exist, it is frequently counterproductive, based on a few lectures and some experience in a group that is run according to an extremely abstinent therapeutic style. Such training may create the impression that the therapist leading a group has little to do but to let the process take its course. But this is certainly not the way to lead IPT-G groups, or any of the other focused and time-limited models of group therapy. Expertise in individual therapy does not confer equal skill in running groups. In fact, it often gets in the way because of the tendency to treat individuals in rotation and to miss important aspects of the group culture that can impede or reinforce effective treatment.

Group psychotherapy training consists of three components. The first of these is a reasonable introduction to group theory, with emphasis on an approach that leads to an understanding of the group system. For the individually trained therapist, the major transition is to appreciate how to understand and use the whole group as the context in which work is being conducted. The second component involves detailed and preferably observed supervision of several groups. This is best done by means of observation windows or video replay; audiotapes, though also used, are less satisfactory. Most powerful learning occurs through doing, not through reading. By working with actual group members, the clinician can learn how to adapt already developed individual strategies for effective use in a group. One effective method is for the novice group therapist to serve as a co-therapist with an experienced group clinician and then to move on to a solo-led group with supervision. The third component of group psychotherapy training is experience as a group member. This experience need not occur in a formal treatment group; indeed, many group organizations offer experiential training groups that will alert the clinician to the nuances of the group experience. In addition, the National Registry of Certified Group Psychotherapists provides a national standard based on a master's-level mental health degree and demonstrated criteria in regard to group training (National Registry of Certified Group Psychotherapists, 1995).

Training in IPT-G

As with individual IPT, no formal training or certification process has been established to determine competence in the delivery of IPT-G. However, we can offer the following suggested guidelines for training in IPT-G: (1) Read this treatment manual. (2) Participate in a formal workshop or course at an established IPT-G training facility. (3) Review group transcripts or view IPT-G videotapes at an established IPT-G training facility. And (4) from an IPT-G expert, receive detailed supervision of at least one completed IPT-G group.

In addition, those wishing to apply IPT-G for research purposes are advised to contact Denise E. Wilfley, Ph.D., in order to establish an appropriate training and monitoring protocol.

Training Centers for Individual IPT in North America

Cornell Psychotherapy Institute
Cornell University Medical College
525 East 68th Street, Room 1322
New York, NY 10021
> *Contact:* John C. Markowitz, M.D. (212-746-3774), or Kathleen F. Clougherty, A.C.S.W. (212-721-2569).

Department of Psychology
University of Iowa
200 Hawkins Drive
Iowa City, IA 52242
   Contact: Scott Stuart, M.D., or Michael O'Hara, Ph.D.
   (319-353-6960).

Interpersonal Therapy Clinic
Clarke Institute
250 College Street
Toronto, Ontario
M5T 1R8 Canada
   Contact: Laurie Gillies, Ph.D. (416-979-6925).

San Diego State University/University of California San Diego Joint
Doctoral Program in Clinical Psychology
6495 Alvarado Road
San Diego, CA 92120
   Contact: Denise E. Wilfley, Ph.D. (619-594-3676), or R. Robinson
   Welch, Ph.D. (619-594-3254).

Western Psychiatric Institute and Clinic
3811 O'Hara Street
Pittsburgh, PA 15213
   Contact: Cleon Cornes, M.D. (412-624-2211).

TRAINING CENTERS FOR IPT-G IN NORTH AMERICA

Virginia Ayres, Ph.D.
Private Practice
Erie, PA 16506
   Contact: Virginia Ayers (814-835-3829, mishka2@erie.net).

San Diego State University/University of California San Diego Joint
Doctoral Program in Clinical Psychology

6495 Alvarado Road
San Diego, CA 92120
  Contact: Denise E. Wilfley, Ph.D.
  (619-594-3254, dwilfley@psychology.sdsu.edu),
  or R.Robinson Welch, Ph.D.(619-594-3254, welch2@mail.sdsu.edu).

University of British Columbia
201-1600 Howe Street
Vancouver, BC V6Z2L9 Canada
  Contact: Roy MacKenzie, M.D.
  (604-822-7669, rmack@interchange.ubc.ca).

THE USE OF IPT-G IN
MENTAL HEALTH SETTINGS

IPT was specifically developed for the treatment of major depression. This is the largest single category of presenting complaint in service systems. The next largest category comprises the range of anxiety disorders, with general anxiety disorder (GAD) the most prevalent of these disorders. GAD is commonly combined with substantial loading of depressive symptoms. Many reactive upset states related to acute stress events also have a large component of depressive symptoms. All service systems report a smaller but still high-service-using cohort of patients with long-standing dysthymic symptoms. In short, the general mental health delivery scene is overwhelmingly concerned with aspects of depression. Groups composed with this population in mind can address a significant proportion of the clinical needs involved, often in conjunction with psychotropic medication. With slight modifications to the protocol, IPT-G groups can successfully be utilized in mental health settings. Several examples follow.

First, IPT-G groups can be employed in an intensive manner in a day treatment program or an inpatient setting where there may be several group meetings each day. Generally such programs are restricted to quite severely dysfunctional patients and consist of a variety of therapeutic components. Although use of this format has not been formally tested, R. Robinson Welch has successfully adapted IPT-G for such a setting. For instance, on admission, patients are encouraged to identify the interpersonal precipitants involved in the exacerbation of their symptoms and/or their hospitalization (e.g., an argument with a spouse or family member, increasing isolation). The therapist uses this information to help patients establish short-term goals that can be worked on in both the group and the ward milieu (e.g., "Identify and share feelings of frustration with my spouse," "Maintain connections with my friends when I am out of the hospital"). During the group sessions, the therapist works to facilitate connections among the members around these universal themes. Within this model, the therapist takes on a more instructional role in assisting patients to find alternative ways to manage the interpersonal issues that are associated with re-hospitalization. A day treatment program could also consider this format augmented by other treatment models such as a cognitive behavior therapy group, art therapy, or a stress management program.

Second, within an outpatient or day treatment program, a brief open-group IPT-G model can address acute situational problems primarily of a reactive nature with a loading of depressive symptoms. Such a group has a constantly changing membership, with a limit on the number of weekly sessions available for any given patient, perhaps a maximum of eight. The group sessions are quite highly structured in this model, involving a focus on each member in turn. The group functions as a reflecting audience, often providing valuable support, encouragement, and practical ideas. Considerable vicarious learning occurs. Group process is kept to a supportive level and is not used in an interpretive manner. Each session ends with a go-around to set practical interpersonal goals to be worked on before the next session. The eight sessions might be scheduled over several months, with increasing spacing as functional competency is restored (MacKenzie, 1997).

Groups of this nature have the limited goal of helping patients get over an immediate distressing period; they do not provide formal psychotherapy. Nevertheless, the principles of IPT serve as the foundation of the group approach. Most of the time is spent dealing with an individual member as the focus of discussion. Generally, patients focus their difficulties on interpersonal triggering incidents, which are addressed in a concrete fashion. The therapists can slant the discussions toward interpersonal problems and can implicitly apply the strategies of the appropriate problem area. The great majority of the members are likely to have issues of loss or interpersonal disputes. Indeed, group composition could be based on these specific problem areas.

This group model, though not subjected to formal outcome measures, has been used for several years in a network of inner-city outpatient departments with overall positive clinical results and good patient satisfaction measures.

Third, IPT-G can be considered for long-term maintenance therapy for depression in a manner analogous to the individual model developed for this purpose. Patients who have experienced even a small number of major depressive episodes and have responded to either pharmacological or psychotherapeutic treatment remain at significant risk for future episodes. Many patients successfully treated with IPT for acute depressive episodes continue to show significant impairment in social adjustment that is considered to increase the patient's vulnerability to recurrence. A number of studies have documented the effectiveness of maintenance sessions conducted on a monthly schedule (e.g., Spanier et al., 1996). The simultaneous use of IPT with medications is well established (Weissman et al., 2000).

A manual has been developed for the purpose of maintenance application known as IPT-M. This approach employs the same focus on problem areas as IPT-G, except that grief is generally not relevant unless a new occurrence of loss occurs during the treatment. Role transitions often take the form of adaptation to a nondepressed state, with a concurrent increase in expectations from others for more active involvement. Interpersonal deficits noted in the acute treatment phase continue to be a major focus, often dealing with characterologic difficulties in the area of avoidant and dependent traits. And interpersonal disputes often have a recurrent presence as the therapeutic focus.

Although group therapy maintenance approaches have not been specifically studied, the overall comparative literature is consistent in finding that individual implementation and group implementation of the same theoretical model for a variety of conditions show no difference in outcome (Piper and Joyce, 1996; McRoberts et al., 1998). There is little reason to doubt that the same would be true of IPT-G. Indeed, the use of a group automatically builds in an interpersonal environment that, if anything, should provide additional specific benefits in terms of reinforcing the principles of IPT.

IMPLEMENTING GROUP PROGRAMS IN MANAGED CARE SETTINGS

In managed care systems there is a constant call for greater use of groups. This circumstance tends to be driven by economic considerations, but without enough attention paid to the organization of group programs. It is common to hear comments about the difficulty involved in implementing greater use of groups. Such comments reflect a failure to fully address larger system-organizational issues. Detailed descriptions of complex group therapy programs have been described elsewhere (MacKenzie, 1995, 1997). As a brief introduction to this complex subject, a compendium of critical implementation strategies is outlined below.

1. Regarding public administrative support, a clear and enthusiastic statement from senior management of the intent to develop group programming sets the stage for possible developments and legitimizes the value of the group modality.
2. The position of group coordinator needs to be established. Programs are unlikely to flourish without such a position with dedicated time. Moderate-sized programs require a half-time commitment, and larger programs entail a full-time commit-

ment. The role of the coordinator is to plan, promote, market, and supervise all groups in an integrated formal program.

3. Planning should be based on an analysis of utilization patterns in terms of presenting disorders, and the groups should be geared toward addressing these through the use of empirically supported models such as IPT and CBT. Planning is best executed on an annual basis, with frequency of groups based on the predicted patient volume for each type of group. Groups are likely to be needed in all three time categories: brief (up to eight sessions), time-limited (up to twenty-four sessions), and longer term (with intensive psychotherapy or maintenance functions). The examples in the preceding section follow this principle.

4. A regular group status sheet should be circulated to all potential referring and assessing sources on a regular basis, probably weekly in large programs.

5. A common intake assessment process should be geared toward making informed group placements. Ideally, this process would be a specialized function within the system, or at least a standardized format for all clinicians to follow. Without this component, the effective use of purpose-designed groups would be difficult. Brief assessments, often conducted over the telephone by relatively naive staff, are generally not satisfactory. The use of simple change-measure questionnaires is encouraged. Indeed, major accrediting organizations are now insisting that such questionnaires be regularly employed. But beyond mandated service documentation, they can also be of use to clinicians in assessing patients and tracking improvement.

6. Some type of consistently employed clinical supervision is essential. Groups have the capacity to pull even experienced therapists off a position of basic neutrality. At the very least, time for all group therapists to meet regularly for peer supervision is needed. The types of groups described in this book are inten-

sive and designed for major psychiatric syndromes that bring with them a substantial level of challenge for the therapist.

7. Basic facilities are required in terms of adequately sized rooms that are kept in good operating condition. Also very helpful are rooms with observation or video transmission capabilities that could be used for unobtrusive clinical supervision purposes by the group coordinator.

8. Program clinical operating arrangements need to be reviewed. Is time allowed for the extra charting and contact functions involved in doing group work? Is there some incentive for using a group format? Does the benefits plan allow for substitution of three group sessions for one individual session? These arrangements may take many forms, ranging from reduction of assessment expectations, to access to continuing education programs, to salary incentives.

Pretherapy Preparation: Information Regarding Group Therapy

This information sheet is intended for people who are about to begin group therapy, or who are considering it as a possible treatment. It is useful when starting group therapy to have some general ideas about how groups help people and how to get the most out of the experience. Group therapy is different from individual therapy in that many helpful events take place among the members and not just between the leader and the members. That is one reason why it is important for all members to receive a general introduction before beginning. Please read this material carefully, and feel free to discuss any part of it with your group leader. The issues raised in this handout are also useful to talk about during the first few sessions in the group.

DO GROUPS REALLY HELP PEOPLE?

Group therapy is widely used and has been a standard part of treatment programs for the last forty to fifty years. Sometimes it is used as the main or perhaps the only treatment approach. This is especially true for outpatients. At other times it is used as part of a treatment approach that may include individual therapy, pharmaceutical drugs, and other activities. Group therapy has been shown in research studies to be an effective treatment. Studies that have compared individual and group approaches indicate that both are about equally effective. The difference with groups, of course, is that a group has to form, and the members need to get to know each other a bit before it can be of the greatest benefit. Most people have participated in some type of nontherapy group—for example, in schools, churches, or community activities. Therapy groups will have many of the same features. The difference is that in a therapy group the leader has a responsibility to ensure that the group stays focused on its treatment goals and that all members participate in this objective.

HOW GROUP THERAPY WORKS

Group therapy is based on the idea that many of the difficulties that people have in their lives can be understood as problems in getting along with other people. As children we learn ways of getting close and talking to others and ways of solving issues with others. Often these early patterns are then applied in adult relationships. Sometimes, however, these ways are not as effective as they might be, despite good intentions. Very often symptoms such as anxiety or unhappiness, bad feelings about yourself, or a general sense of dissatisfaction with life reflect the unsatisfactory state of important relationships in your life. Groups offer an opportunity to learn more about these "interpersonal" patterns.

There are many different kinds of groups. Some are designed to provide members with information about a particular topic, such as eating disorders; others focus on a particular skill, such as assertiveness. Some are quite structured and may use a written manual, as in cognitive-behavioral groups; others focus on understanding more about yourself and the nature of your important relationships. No matter what kind of group you are in, this information sheet is designed to let you know about how groups work and how you can get the most from your group experience.

COMMON MYTHS ABOUT
GROUP THERAPY

1. Although it is true that groups offer an efficient way of treating several people at once, group therapy is not a second-rate treatment in the sense that it has less power to help people than other treatments. As mentioned above, studies show that most of the "talking therapies" are about equally effective.

2. Some people are concerned that a therapy group will be like a forced confessional where they have to reveal all of the details of their life. This is not the case. Instead of discussing specific details, members tend to talk about the patterns in relationships and the meanings these have for them. As they become more familiar with each other and begin to trust each other, they find their own level of comfort regarding how much they want to disclose about their personal lives. Details about where you live or work, even your last name, are therefore not necessary for effective involvement in the group.

3. Some people worry that being in a room with other people with difficulties will make everyone worse off. This idea of "the blind leading the blind" is understandable, but in practice people find that the process of talking about their problems is very helpful. Indeed, finding out that others have had similar problems can be reassuring. Many group therapy patients are surprised to discover that they have something to offer to other people.

4. Some media presentations of group therapy suggest that people often lose control in groups and become so upset that they can't function or so angry that they act destructively. In reality, however, such outcomes are very rare. In any case, the group therapist has been trained to remain alert and responsible, and to calm things down if the tension gets too high.

5. When picturing themselves in a therapy group, some people find themselves feeling concerned that they may be rejected or excluded by other group members, that they may be judged harshly by the others, or that they may lose their sense of themselves and be carried along by the group to a place where they don't wish to go. All of

these fears are perfectly understandable; indeed, almost everyone experiences them to some extent when they enter any new social group situation. It is good to talk about such fears early in the group so that they can be acknowledged, understood, and then put behind you.

HOW TO GET THE MOST OUT OF GROUP

1. The more you can involve yourself in the group, the more you will get out of it. In particular, try to identify the sorts of things that you find upsetting or bothersome. Try to be as open and honest as possible in what you say. Group time is precious; it is a time to be working on serious issues, not just passing the time of day. Listen hard to what people are saying, think through what they mean, and try to make sense of it. You can help others by letting them know what you make of what they say and how it affects you. Many of the issues talked about in groups are general human matters with which we can all identify. At the same time, listen hard to what others say to you about your part in the group. This process of learning from others is an important way to gain from the group experience. It takes time to appreciate how much a group can help you. So it is important that you commit yourself to attend a few sessions of the group before deciding if it's worthwhile for you. Before the group starts, talk with your therapist about what the expectations are in terms of the length of your particular group.

2. One way of thinking about group is to view it as a "living laboratory" of relationships. It is a place where you can try out new ways of talking to people, a place to take some risks. You are a responsible member of the group and can help to make it an effective experience for everybody. A good way to think about how a group can help people is this. Consider a person risking a different way of talking about personal matters, getting a response from the other members that confirms that it sounds all right, and then trying to make sense of the experience.

3. Do your best to translate your inner reactions into words. Group is not a "tea party" where everything has to be done in a socially

proper fashion. It is a place to try to explore the meaning of what goes on and the reactions inside that get stirred up.

4. Remember that how people talk is as important as what they say. As you listen to others and as you think about what you yourself have been saying, try to think beyond the words to the other messages being sent. Sometimes the meaning of the words does not match the tone of voice or the expression on the face.

5. Because the group is a place to learn from the experience itself, it is important to focus upon what is happening inside the group room among the members and between each member and the leader. Often, understanding these group relationships throws new light on outside relationships. Many people have found it helpful to think about themselves in terms of the things they know and don't know about themselves, and the things that others know or don't know.

Table A.1 outlines these group relationships. One of the tasks in group is to try to enlarge the box labeled "PUBLIC KNOWLEDGE" through three main methods: first, by talking about things that you normally keep hidden about yourself or speaking about your thoughts concerning others (self-disclosure); second, by listening to what others are saying about what might be your blind spots (receiving feedback); and, third, by making a genuine attempt to understand more about yourself (personal insight).

COMMON
STUMBLING BLOCKS

1. It is normal to feel anxiety about being in groups. Almost everyone experiences it to some extent. One way of dealing with it is to talk about it at an early point in the group. (This is a good model of the usefulness of talking about things so that they can be clarified and the anxiety related to them can be reduced.)

2. It is the role of the leader to encourage members to talk with each other and to help keep the group focused on important tasks. The leader is not there to supply ready answers to specific problems. One

TABLE A.1   Group Relationships

	Things I DO know about myself	Things I do NOT know about myself	
Things others DO know about me	PUBLIC KNOWLEDGE	Receive feedback	BLIND SPOTS
Things others do NOT know about me	Self-disclosure HIDDEN SELF	Personal insight	UNKNOWN SELF

of the things you will experience in group is learning to benefit from the process of talking with other people and not just getting pat answers.

3. Try hard to put into words the connection between how you are reacting or feeling and what is happening between you and other people both in the group and outside. It is all right to be emotional. This process of trying to understand reactions or symptoms in terms of relationships is important.

4. Many group members find themselves experiencing a sense of puzzlement or discouragement after the excitement of the first few group sessions. Please live through this stage. It almost always occurs, and it reflects the fact that groups need time to develop their full benefit for the members. Once the group has gotten past this stage, it is in a much stronger position to be helpful.

5. From time to time in the group you may find yourself experiencing such negative feelings as disappointment, frustration, or even anger. It is important to talk about these reactions in a constructive fashion. Many people have difficulty with managing such feelings, and it is part of the group's task to examine them. Sometimes negative feelings may be directed toward the leader. It is equally important that these be talked about as well.

6. Try hard to apply what you learn in group to outside situations. Many group members have found it very useful to talk to the group about how they might apply what they are learning, then try it out in their personal lives and report back to the group about how it went. Studies have shown that the more you can do this, the more likely therapy will become "real" and the more you will get out of it. Many people report that keeping a regular personal journal is helpful in terms of keeping on track with important issues between sessions. Remember that the rest of the world does not necessarily run the same way as a therapy group. Try out your ideas in the group first to test whether your plans are well thought out.

7. Many people come to therapy groups because things have not been going well in their lives. There is a temptation to take the first advice you hear and then decide to make a big change. But please wait so that you have a chance to think about your ideas and talk about them in the group before making important life decisions.

GROUP EXPECTATIONS

1. *Confidentiality*: It is very important to make sure that things that are talked about in the group do not get talked about outside. You may, of course, want to discuss your experience with people close to you, but even then it is important not to attach names or specific information to the talk. In our experience, breaks in confidentiality have been extremely uncommon. Please be sure that you don't talk about others outside the group, just as you don't want them to talk about you.

2. *Attendance and punctuality*: It is very important that you attend all sessions and arrive on time. Once a group gets going, it functions as a group, and even if just one member is absent, it is not the same. So for your own sake and for the sake of all of the members, please be a regular attendee. If for some reason it is impossible for you to make a session, then call in advance and discuss it with your therapist or at least leave some information about the reason for your absence. In

this way the group will know you are not coming and won't find it-self waiting to get down to work until you arrive. In the case of out-patient groups, it is useful for members to spend some time periodically talking about major absences such as trips or vacations and to discuss how to plan for these as a group.

3. *Socializing with other group members*: It is important to think of group as a treatment setting and not as a replacement for other social activities. Group members are strongly advised not to have outside contacts with each other. The reason for this is that if you have a spe-cial relationship with another group member, that relationship may interfere with your getting the most out of the group interaction. The two of you would find yourselves having secrets from the group or not addressing issues because of your friendship. If you do have out-side contacts with group members, it is important that you talk about them in the group so that the effects of these contacts can be taken into account. Indeed, you are asked to make a commitment to report such contacts within the group. (Note: Some groups that deal with learning and applying social skills may encourage members to prac-tice such skills together.)

4. *Contact between group sessions*: Except in truly urgent circum-stances, the therapist does not generally expect to have contact with group members outside of the group itself. All such contacts will be considered as part of the larger frame of the group experience, and the therapist may bring this material back into the group sessions. In addition, it is generally advisable not to engage in any other regular therapy while in the group, with the exception of seeing your doctor for medication management. Any concerns or plans about seeing other therapists need to be discussed with the group leader before the group begins.

5. *Alcohol or drugs*: The group is a place for sensitive personal dis-cussions, so it is important that you not come to a session under the influence of alcohol or drugs (except prescription medicines). The point here is not that it is good or bad to use alcohol or drugs but, rather, that they get in the way of making the most of the group ex-perience. As a general rule, you will be asked to leave the session if

your behavior is significantly affected. Nor are food, beverages, or smoking allowed in the group room, as these tend to distract from the work of the group.

This material was adapted from "Time-Managed Group Psychotherapy: Effective Clinical Applications," by Dr. K. Roy MacKenzie (American Psychiatric Press, Inc., 1997). Permission is granted for it to be reprinted for clinical use.

APPENDIX B

Descriptions of
Commonly Used
Assessment Questionnaires

QUESTIONNAIRES FOR COMPLETION
BY THE PATIENT

SYMPTOMS

Symptom Checklist (SCL-90-R). This ninety-item, self-report symptom inventory is the latest version of the original psychological symptom portion of the Cornell Medical Index. There is a high degree of correlation between the SCL-90-R subscale scores and comparable Minnesota Multiphasic Personality Inventory dimensions. Results are expressed on nine symptom dimensions: somatization, obsessive-compulsive, interpersonal sensitivity, depression, anxiety, hostility, phobic anxiety, paranoid ideation, and psychoticism. A Global Seventy Index gives an overall measure of symptom status. This is the most widely used standard measure of general psychopathology.

National Computer Systems Assessments
P.O. Box 1416

Minneapolis, Minnesota 55440
Telephone: 800-627-7271

Brief Symptom Inventory (BSI).   This is a fifty-three-item brief version
of the SCL-90 with the same nine symptom dimensions.

National Computer Systems Assessments
P.O. Box 1416
Minneapolis, Minnesota 55440
Telephone: 800-627-7271

Outcome Questionnaire (OQ-45).   This forty-five-item questionnaire
was designed for use in service settings. In addition to an overall total score, it features subscale scores concerning symptoms, interpersonal functioning, and social functioning.

American Professional Credentialing Services LLC
10421 Stevenson Road, P.O. Box 346
Stevenson, Maryland 21153-0346
Telephone: 500-488-2727
Fax: 410-329-3777

Beck Depression Inventory (BDI).   This twenty-one-item questionnaire
covers the major features of major depressive disorder. It is the standard measure for patient self-reports of depression and can be used
sequentially to track response to treatment.

The Psychological Corporation
555 Academic Court
San Antonio, Texas 78204-2498
Telephone: 800-634-0424

Emotional Eating Scale (EES).   The Emotional Eating Scale (Arnow,
Kenardy, and Agras, 1995), which assesses the urge to cope with neg-

ative affect by eating, features a list of emotions that cluster into anger/frustration, anxiety, and depression subscales. It has been shown to provide an assessment of antecedents to binge eating for clinical populations.

Eating Disorder Examination (EDE). The EDE (Fairburn and Cooper, 1993) is an investigator-based interview designed to assess the main behavioral and attitudinal aspects of eating disorders. This interview provides a detailed assessment of the degree of dietary restraint, of such key behaviors as binge eating and inappropriate compensatory purging, and of concerns about thinness, weight, and eating.

Eating Disorder Examination Questionnaire (EDE-Q). The EDE-Q was designed to provide a self-report version of the EDE interview that could be completed in less than fifteen minutes (Fairburn and Beglin, 1994). To parallel the EDE interview, the EDE-Q focuses on a patient's past twenty-eight days to assess the main behavioral and attitudinal features of his or her eating disorder. It uses similar probe questions and a similar rating scheme, although it does not include any of the key definitions provided in the interview. The EDE-Q also assesses frequencies of key behavioral features in terms of the *number of days* on which particular forms of behavior occur rather than the *number of individual episodes,* because there is evidence with respect to binge eating that this method is more accurate.

INTERPERSONAL FUNCTIONING

Inventory of Interpersonal Problems (IIP). This questionnaire deals with interpersonal problems, and the wording of its questions is particularly well suited to a clinical population. The question stems are either "It is hard for me to (be assertive)" or "I am too (controlling)." It contains sixty-four items, but a thirty-two-item version is also available. The IIP measures eight problem clusters that form a circumplex pattern based on the two major axes of Dominance and

Nurturance (Alden, Wiggins, and Pincus, 1990). A vector is calculated in order to achieve the best representation of the two-dimensional space. In addition, conflict scores are calculated for each of the four pairs of opposite segments. A positive conflict score indicates that the patient has an elevated score on conceptually opposite qualities such as Dominance and Submission. The interpersonal trait measures of Extraversion and Agreeableness can also be plotted on the circle.

The Psychological Corporation
555 Academic Court
San Antonio, Texas 78204-2498
Telephone: 800-634-0424

Analysis of Social Behavior (SASB). This instrument is based on a unique circumplex model of interpersonal functioning (Benjamin, 1974) that comprises two axes. The first axis runs from positive Affiliation (loving, approaching) to negative Affiliation (attacking, rejecting), whereas the other goes from high Independence (autonomy) to high Interdependence (enmeshment). This conceptual space may be applied to relationships (how one acts on the other, and how one reacts to the other) or to a view of one's self (introject). The measure can be applied to Best/Worst/Ideal views of self as well as to specific intimate relationships drawn from the patient's life over time. These might include mother, father, and the parental relationship itself as experienced during the preadolescent years. A full assessment of significant figures usually entails eight relationships, which add up to 288 items. The SASB provides a view of specific relationship patterns rather than a global description of personality dimensions.

Dr. Lorna Benjamin
Department of Psychology
University of Utah
Salt Lake City, Utah 84112
Telephone: 601-581-4463

Social Functioning

Medical Outcomes Study Short Form (SF-36). This thirty-six-item questionnaire was designed to assess general functioning at repeated intervals.

Social Adjustment Scale. The Social Adjustment Scale (Weissman and Bothwell, 1976) is a measure of social behavior that has been widely used to assess actual interpersonal functioning. It provides scores for different role areas (e.g., family and work) and is sensitive to change resulting from psychotherapy.

UCLA Loneliness Scale—Revised. The UCLA Loneliness Scale—Revised (Russell, Peplau, and Cutrona, 1980), which measures perceptions of loneliness or inadequacy in social relationships, can be used to determine the degree of current interpersonal deficits.

Personality Traits

NEO Personality Inventory (NEO-PI). This 181-item instrument is a widely used measure of personality traits that appear to have the same structure in both a normal population and a personality disordered population; only the extent of the behaviors is different. The five-factor solution consists of Neuroticism, Extraversion, Openness, Agreeableness, and Conscientiousness. Each dimension has several facets based on item subsets (Costa and Widiger, 1994).

QUESTIONNAIRES FOR COMPLETION BY THE CLINICIAN

General Assessment

Global Assessment of Functioning (GAF). This questionnaire is available through the American Psychiatric Association in connection with the *Diagnostic and Statistical Manual of Mental Disorders, Fourth*

Edition (DSM-IV) (Washington, D.C.: American Psychiatric Association, 1994).

Demographics/Statistics

Listed on the registration sheet for each patient are basic demographic data including age, sex, marital status, education, and employment status. Also listed, when possible, are data concerning the patient's use of both health and mental health services before and after treatment, as such data provide a powerful measure of effectiveness.

Group Process Measures

Group Climate Questionnaire (GCQ).   This twelve-item questionnaire, designed to be completed by group members, describes the overall group atmosphere.

Dr. K. Roy MacKenzie, M.D.
201-1600 Howe Street
Vancouver, B.C. V6Z 2L9 Canada
Fax: 604-669-7783
E-mail: rmack@interchange.ubc.ca

California Psychotherapy Alliance Scales (CALPAS-G).   Available in twelve- and twenty-four-item versions, this scale is completed by group members to address their own relationship to the group.

Alliance Scales

Langley Porter Psychiatric Institute
Box F-0984
University of California
401 Parnassus Avenue
San Francisco, California 94143-0984
Telephone: 415-476-7562

APPENDIX C

Pretreatment Fact Sheet

Facts About Binge
Eating Disorder

Binge eating disorder is a newly recognized eating disorder that probably affects millions of Americans. People with binge eating disorder frequently eat large amounts of food while feeling a loss of control over their eating. This disorder is different from binge-purge syndrome (bulimia nervosa) in that people with binge eating disorder usually do not purge afterward by vomiting or using laxatives. Binge eating disorder is an eating disorder that requires specialized and focused treatment.

1. *How does someone know if he or she has binge eating disorder?*

Most of us overeat from time to time, and many people feel that they frequently eat more than they should. Eating large amounts of food, however, does not mean that someone has binge eating disorder. *Men and women with binge eating disorder experience the following:*

- Frequent episodes of eating what others would consider an abnormally large amount of food.
- Frequent feelings of being unable to control what or how much is being eaten.
- Several of these behaviors or feelings: (a) eating much more rapidly than usual; (b) eating until feeling uncomfortably full;

(c) eating large amounts of food, even when not physically hungry; (d) feelings of disgust, depression, or guilt after overeating.

2. *How common is binge eating disorder, and who is at risk?*

Although binge eating disorder has only recently been recognized as a distinct condition, it is probably the most common eating disorder. Most people with binge eating disorder are obese (i.e., more than 20 percent above a healthy body weight), but normal-weight people can also be affected. Binge eating disorder probably affects 2 percent of all adults, or about 1–2 million Americans. Among mildly obese people in self-help or commercial weight loss programs, 10 to 15 percent have binge eating disorder. The disorder is even more common in those with severe obesity.

Binge eating disorder is slightly more common among women, with three women affected for every two men. The disorder affects African Americans as often as Caucasians; its frequency in other ethnic groups is not yet known. Obese people with binge eating disorder often become overweight at a younger age than those without the disorder. They also have more frequent episodes of losing and regaining weight (yo-yo dieting).

3. *Do individuals with binge eating disorder struggle with their weight?*

Men and women with binge eating disorder have struggled with *repeated failures at weight loss* (repeated weight losses followed by weight gains). Not only does the binge eating lead to weight gain, but it is often followed by a vicious cycle of dieting and binge eating.

4. *What is the aim of this treatment program?*

Different than other traditional weight loss programs, this treatment program is designed to treat your eating disorder. Treatment is structured to help you decrease and eliminate your problems with binge eating, which, in turn, should have an effect on your weight.

5. *How will this treatment program affect my weight?*

Research data show that when people with binge eating disorder stop bingeing they are more successful at regulating their weight. That is, when people with binge eating disorder stop bingeing (stop eating large amounts of food while feeling a loss of control over eating), they are often more successful at stabilizing their weight and losing weight.

6. *How will interpersonal psychotherapy help ease my problems with binge eating?*

Men and women with binge eating disorder often describe themselves as "stress eaters." Indeed, according to reports by persons with binge eating disorder, negative feelings are the most frequent trigger for binge eating. Interpersonal therapy will help you learn to deal more effectively with negative emotions and relationship difficulties that may lead to "stress-induced" binge eating. By learning to identify, manage, and express your reactions and feelings, you will be less likely to turn to food to soothe and comfort you. That is, by developing a better relationship with yourself (learning to tune in and identify what you are feeling as opposed to numbing yourself with food) and by developing better relationships with others, you will become less likely to use food as a way to manage your negative feelings. The better able you are to manage your feelings and your relationships with others, the more successful you will be at eliminating your problems with binge eating.

7. *Why am I being asked not to participate in a commercial weight loss program while I am receiving this treatment?*

Commercial weight loss programs are not designed to treat people with eating disorders. For this reason they cannot address the unique and special concerns of men and women with binge eating disorder. Indeed, people who struggle with binge eating disorder typically consider themselves to be "diet program drop-outs." Most people with binge eating disorder have tried a series of different types of programs with only limited long-term success. In fact, the experience of undergoing one of these programs often leaves persons with binge eating disorder feeling like they are failures and saying to themselves "If only I had more 'will power' I would have been successful." We believe that attempts at weight management will meet with limited long-term success until the problems with binge eating are under control.

8. Since I won't be in a commercial weight loss program, what can I do on my own to manage my weight?

The focus of this treatment program is to eliminate your problems with binge eating. By tackling your problem with binge eating, you will begin to normalize and stabilize your eating patterns, which should affect your weight. Data do suggest that people who stop binge eating are more successful at stabilizing their weight and losing weight. Further, by beginning to feel better about yourself (which is an added benefit of stopping the binge eating), you will gradually begin to take more time out for yourself to engage in behaviors that are compatible with a healthy lifestyle and successful weight management (such as moderate exercise, heart-healthy eating, and so on).

References

Agras, W. S., Walsh, B. T., Fairburn, C. G., Wilson, G. T., Kraemer, H. C. (in press). A multicenter comparison of cognitive-behavioral therapy and interpersonal psychotherapy for bulimia nervosa. *Arch. Gen. Psychiatry.*

Alden, L. E., Wiggins, J. S., and Pincus, A. L. (1990). Construction of circumplex scales for the Inventory of Interpersonal Problems. *Journal of Personality Assessment, 55,* 521–536.

American Psychiatric Association (1994). *Diagnostic and Statistical Manual of Mental Disorders, 4th ed.* Washington, D.C.: American Psychiatric Association.

Angus, L., and Gillies, L. A. (1994). Counseling the borderline client: An interpersonal approach. *Canadian Journal of Counseling, 28*(1), 69–82.

Arnow, B., Kenardy, J., and Agras, W. S. (1995). The emotional eating scale: The development of a measure to assess coping with negative affect by eating. *International Journal of Eating Disorders, 18* (1), 79-90.

Beck, A. T., Rush, A. J., Shaw, B. F., and Emery, G. (1979). *Cognitive Therapy of Depression.* New York: Guilford Press.

Benjamin, L. S. (1974). Structural analysis of social behavior. *Psychological Review, 81,* 392-425.

Bowlby, J. (1982). *Attachment and Loss: Vol. 1. Attachment,* 2nd ed. New York: Basic Books.

Carroll, K. M., and Nuro, K. F. (1997). The use and development of manuals. In K. M. Carrol (Ed.), *Improving Compliance with Alcoholism Treatment.* NIAAA Project MATCH Monograph Series, Vol. 6 (pp. 53–72). NIH Publication 97-143. Bethesda, Md.: National Institute on Alcohol Abuse and Alcoholism.

Costa, P. T., and Widiger, T. A. (Eds.). (1994). *Personality Disorders and the Five-Factor Model of Personality.* Washington, D.C.: American Psychological Association.

Dies, R. R. (1994). The therapist's role in group treatments. In H. S. Bernard and K. R. MacKenzie (Eds.), *Basics of Group Psychotherapy.* New York: Guilford Press.

Fairburn, C. G. (1998). Interpersonal psychotherapy for bulimia nervosa. In J. C. Markowitz (ed.), *Interpersonal psychotherapy* (pp. 99–128). Washington, D.C.: American Psychiatric Press.

Fairburn, C. G., and Beglin, S. J. (1994). Assessment of eating disorders: Interview or self-report questionnaire? *International Journal of Eating Disorders, 16,* 363-370.

Fairburn, C. G., and Cooper, Z. (1993). The eating disorder examination (12th ed.). In C. G. Fairburn and G. T. Wilson (Eds.), Binge eating: assessment and treatment. New York: Guilford Press.

Fairburn, C. G., Jones, R., Peveler, R. C., Carr, S. J., Solomon, R. A., O'Connor, M. E., Burton, J., and Hope, R. A. (1991). Three psychological treatments for bulimia nervosa. *Archives of General Psychiatry, 48,* 463–469.

Fairburn, C. G., Jones, R., Peveler, R. C., Hope, R. A., and O'Connor, M. (1993). Psychotherapy and bulimia nervosa: The longer-term effects of interpersonal psychotherapy, behavior therapy and cognitive behavior therapy. *Archives of General Psychiatry, 50,* 419–428.

Fairburn, C. G., Norman, P. A., Welch, S. L., and O'Connor, M. E. (1995). A prospective study of outcome in bulimia nervosa and the long-term effects of three psychological treatments. *Archives of General Psychiatry, 52*(4), 304–312.

Foley, S. H., Rounsaville, B. J., Weissman, M. M., Sholomskas, D., and Chevron, E. (1989). Individual versus conjoint interpersonal psychotherapy for depressed patients with marital disputes. *International Journal of Family Psychiatry, 10,* 29–42.

Frank, E. (1991). Interpersonal psychotherapy as a maintenance treatment for patients with recurrent depression. *Psychotherapy, 28*(2), 259–266.

Frank, E., Kupfer, D. J., Gibbons, R., Hedeker, D., Houch, P. (1999). Interpersonal and social rhythm therapy prevents depressive symptomatology in bipolar patients. Paper presented at the third International Conference on Bipolar Disorder, Pittsburgh, PA.

Frank, E., Kupfer, D. J., Perel, T. M., Cornes, C. L., Jarrett, D. J., Maillinger, A., Thase, M. E., McEachran, A. B., Grochocinski, V. J. (1990). Three year outcomes for maintenance therapies in recurrent depressions, *Arch. Gen. Psychiatry* 47: 1093–1099.

Frank, E., Kupfer, D. J., Wagner, E. F., McEachran, A. B., and Cornes, C. (1991). Efficacy of interpersonal psychotherapy as a maintenance treatment of recurrent depression. *Archives of General Psychiatry, 48,* 1053–1059.

Frank, J. D. (1973). *Persuasion and healing: A comparative study of psychotherapy.* Baltimore: Johns Hopkins University Press.

Gabbard, G. O. (1995). *Psychodynamic Psychiatry in Clinical Practice.* Washington, D.C.: American Psychiatric Press, Inc.

Kaul, T. J., and Bednar, R. L. (1994). Pretraining and structure: Parallel lines yet to meet. In A. Fuhriman and G. M. Burlingame (Eds.), *Handbook of Group Psychotherapy: An Empirical and Clinical Synthesis* (pp. 155–188). New York: Wiley.

Klerman, G. L., Weissman, M. M., Rounsaville, B. J., and Chevron, E. S. (1984). *Interpersonal Psychotherapy of Depression.* New York: Basic Books.

Krupnick, J. L. (in press). *Interpersonal psychotherapy for PTSD following interpersonal trauma: Directions in psychiatry.* New York: The Heatherleigh Co.

Lipsitz, J. D., Fyer, A. J., Markowitz, J. C., and Cherry, S. (1999). An open trial of interpersonal psychotherapy for social phobia. *American Journal of Psychiatry, 156,* 1814–1816.

MacKenzie, K. R. (1994a). The developing structure of the therapy group system. In H. S. Bernard and K. R. MacKenzie (Eds.), *Basics of Group Psychotherapy* (pp. 35–59). New York: Guilford Press.

MacKenzie, K.R. (1995). Rationale for group psychotherapy in managed care. In K.R. MacKenzie (Ed.), *Effective use of group therapy in managed care*. Washington, DC: American Psychiatric Press.

_____. (1994b). Group development. In A. Fuhriman and G. M. Burlingame (Eds.), *Handbook of Group Psychotherapy: An Empirical and Clinical Synthesis* (pp. 223–268). New York: Wiley.

_____. (1997). *Time-Managed Group Psychotherapy: Effective Clinical Applications*. Washington, D.C.: American Psychiatric Press.

Markowitz, J. C. (1994). Psychotherapy of dysthymia. *American Journal of Psychiatry, 151*(8), 1114–1121.

Markowitz, J. C., Kocsis, J. H., Fishman, B., Spielman, L. A., Jacobsberg, L. B., Frances, A. J., Klerman, G. L., and Perry, S. W. (1998). Treatment of depressive symptoms in human immunodeficiency virus-positive patients. *Archives of General Psychiatry, 55*(5), 452–457.

McKay, M., and Paleg, K. (Eds.). (1992). *Focal Group Psychotherapy*. Oakland, Calif.: New Harbinger.

McKenzie, J., McIntosh, V. V., Jordan, J., Joyce, P., Carter, F., Luty, S., and Bulik, C. (1999, April). Interpersonal psychotherapy for anorexia nervosa. Session presented at the 4th International Conference on Eating Disorders, London.

McRoberts, C., Burlingame, G. M., and Hoag, M. J. (1998). *Group Dynamics: Theory, Research, and Practice, 2,* 101–117.

Meyer, A. (1957). *Psychobiology: A Science of Man*. Springfield, Ill.: Charles C. Thomas.

Mufson, L., Weissman, M. M., Moreau, D., Garfinkel, R. (1999). Efficacy of interpersonal psychotherapy for depressed adolescents. *Arch. Gen. Psychiatry* 56: 573–579.

Oei, T. P. S., and Kazmierczak, T. (1997). Factors associated with dropout in a group cognitive behaviour therapy for mood disorders. *Behaviour Research and Therapy, 35*(11), 1025–1030.

Parsons, T. (1951). Illness and the role of the physician: a sociological perspective. *American Journal of Orthopsychiatry, 21,* 452-460.

Piper, W. E., and Joyce, A. S. (1996). A consideration of factors influencing the utilization of time-limited, short-term group therapy. *International Journal of Group Psychotherapy, 46,* 311–328.

Reynolds, C. F., Frank, E., Dew, M. A., Houck, P. R., Miller, M., Mazumdar, S., Perel, J. M., Kuper, D. J. (1999). Treatment of 70+-year-olds with recurrent depression: Excellent short-term but brittle long-term response. *Am. J. Geriatr. Psychiatry* 7:1, 64–69.

Roller, B., and Nelson, V. (1993). Cotherapy. In H. I. Kaplan and B. J. Sadock (Eds.), *Comprehensive Group Psychotherapy,* 3rd ed. (pp. 304–312). Baltimore: Williams and Wilkins.

Russell, D., Peplau, L. A., and Cutrona, C. E. (1980). The revised UCLA loneliness scale: Concurrent and discriminant validity evidence. *Journal of Personality and Social Psychology, 39*(3), 472-480.

Scott, J., and Ikkos, G. (1996). A pilot study of interpersonal psychotherapy for the treatment of chronic somatization in primary care. Paper presented at the First Congress of the World Council of Psychotherapy, Vienna, Austria.

Shapiro, D. A., and Shapiro, D. (1982). Meta-analysis of comparative therapy outcome studies: A replication and refinement. *Psychological Bulletin, 92*, 581–604.

Smith, M. L., Glass, G. V., and Miller, T. I. (1980). *The Benefits of Psychotherapy.* Baltimore: Johns Hopkins University Press.

Spanier, C., and Frank, E. (1998). Maintenance interpersonal psychotherapy: A preventive treatment for depression. In J. C. Markowitz (Ed.), *Interpersonal Psychotherapy* (pp. 67–97). Washington, D.C.: American Psychiatric Press.

Spanier, C., Frank, E., McEachran, A. B., Grochocinski, V. J., and Kupfer, D. J. (1996). The prophylaxis of depressive episodes in recurrent depression following discontinuation of drug therapy: Integrating psychological and biological factors. *Psychological Medicine, 26*, 461–475.

Stuart, S. (1999). Interpersonal psychotherapy for postpartum depression. In L. Miller (Ed.), *Postpartum Psychiatric Disorders* (pp. 143–162). Washington, D.C.: American Psychiatric Press.

Suchman, E. A. (1965a). Social patterns of illness and medical care. *Journal of Health Behavior, 6*, 2–16.

_____. (1965b). Stages of illness and medical care. *Journal of Health Behavior, 6*, 114–128.

Sullivan, H. S. (1953). *The Interpersonal Theory of Psychiatry.* New York: W. W. Norton.

Swartz, H. A., and Markowitz, J. C. (1998). Interpersonal psychotherapy for the treatment of depression in HIV-positive men and women. In J. C. Markowitz (Ed.), *Interpersonal Psychotherapy* (pp. 129–155). Washington, D.C.: American Psychiatric Press.

Tillitski, C. J. (1990). A meta-analysis of estimated effect size for group vs. individual vs. control treatments. *International Journal of Group Psychotherapy, 40*, 215–224.

Tschuschke, V., and Dies, R. R. (1997). The contribution of feedback to outcome in long-term psychotherapy. *Group, 21*(1), 3–15.

Tschuschke, V., MacKenzie, K. R., Haaser, B., and Janke, G. (1996). Self-disclosure, feedback, and outcome in long-term inpatient psychotherapy groups. *Journal of Psychotherapy Practice and Research, 5*(1), 35–44.

_____. (1996b). Body dysmorphic disorder: A cognitive behavior model and pilot randomized controlled trial. *Behavior Research and Therapy, 34*(9), 717–729.

Waltz, J., Addis, M. E., Koerner, K., and Jacobson, N. S. (1993). Testing the integrity of a psychotherapy model protocol: Assessment of adherence and competence. *Journal of Consulting Clinical Psychology, 61*, 620–630.

Weissman, M. M. (1995a). *Mastering Depression: A Patient's Guide to Interpersonal Psychotherapy.* Albany, New York: Graywind Publications.

_____. (1995b). *Patient Assessment Forms Workbook for Interpersonal Psychotherapy Program for Depression*. Albany, N.Y.: Graywind Publications.

Weissman, M. M. and Bothwell, S. (1976). Assessment of social adjustment by patient self-report. *Archives of General Psychiatry, 40,* 1111-1115.

Weissman, M. M., Markowitz, J. C., and Klerman, G. L. (2000). *Comprehensive Guide to Interpersonal Psychotherapy*. Albany, New York: Basic Books.

Wilfley, D. E. (1999, April). Treatment of binge eating disorder: Research findings and clinical applications. In B. T. Walsh (Chair), *Integrating Research and Clinical Practice*. Plenary session presented at the meeting of the 4th International Conference on Eating Disorders, London.

Wilfley, D. E., Agras, W. S., Telch, C. F., Rossiter, E. M., Schneider, J. A., Cole, A. G., Sifford, L., and Raeburn, S. D. (1993). Group cognitive-behavioral therapy and group interpersonal psychotherapy for the nonpurging bulimic: A controlled comparison. *Journal of Consulting and Clinical Psychology, 61,* 296–305.

Wilfley, D. E., Frank, M. A., Welch, R., Spurrell, E. B., and Rounsaville, B. J. (1998). Adapting interpersonal psychotherapy to a group format (IPT-G) for binge eating disorder: Toward a model for adapting empirically supported treatments. *Psychotherapy Research, 8,* 379–391

Wilfley, D. E., Welch, R. R., Stein, R. I., Saelens, B. E., Dounchis, J. Z., and Matt, J. E. (1999, November). The psychological treatment of BED: A controlled comparison of CBT and IPT. Presented at the Eating Disorders Research Society. San Diego, California.

Yalom, I. D. (1995). *The Theory and Practice of Group Psychotherapy,* 4th ed. New York: Basic Books.

Index